Myths, Mysteries and Benefits of Herbs and Essential Oils

Herbs and Essential Oils for the Texas Massage Therapist

Carolyn Gibson

DEDICATION

This is dedicated to Odena Brannam of Lavender Hill Herb Farm,
considered to be the grandmother of herbs in Texas. She was gracious
enough to share her time and knowledge when I was young, inexperienced
and passionate to learn about herbs. I thank her for sharing her recipe for
making Comfrey Oil.
She was in her 80's when she took me under her wing and went to be with
the Lord at the age of 93.

Table of Contents

Carolyn Gibson

NOTE TO READER

This book is meant to be a manual for my CE classes for Texas Massage Therapists. Check out my web site for other classes and schedules.
http://www.TexasMassageTherapsitCEU.com

If you are a Massage Instructor or CE Provider you can contact me for bulk prices on this book. 903 833 1024

You may find recipes and formulas repeated. I have inserted these in chapters when appropriate but have dedicated a chapter for recipes and a chapter for formulas to make it easier for you to find when you start searching for them.

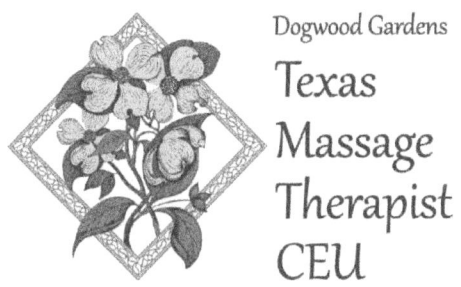

Dogwood Gardens
Texas
Massage
Therapist
CEU

Carolyn Gibson

Disclaimer:

1 Introduction

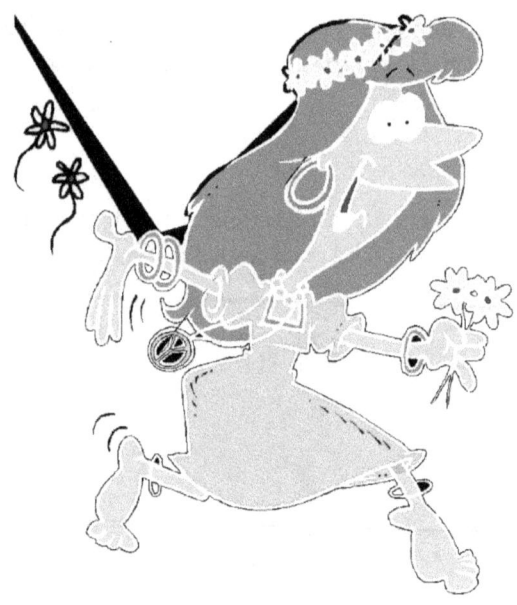

Back in the early 70's there were no Whole Foods or other natural food stores around the corner. A free seminar at SMU on organic farming and herbs was the beginning of my education. I went to a local head shop for whole wheat flour, and what little herbs the shop offered. This was also where I found my first book about massage as a therapeutic benefit and not as a massage parlor treat.

I had already seen the effectiveness of massage on my husband who had been wounded in Vietnam. He had lost 60% use of his hand from nerve damage from a wound in Vietnam   Massage therapist know massage is a natural instinct for healing. With no knowledge of massage, I instinctively massaged my husband's hand whenever we sat watching TV at night. He had yearly exams through the Veterans Administration. The nerves that had been damaged had grown one inch by the time he died in a construction accident.

I have the first issue of Mother Earth News. I subscribed to Herb Companion and the Herb Quarterly. I bought many, many books on herbs. Herbs became like collecting baseball cards. At one time I was growing over 100 different herbs. I would read how healing a particular herb was and run out and get it to grow and make tinctures.

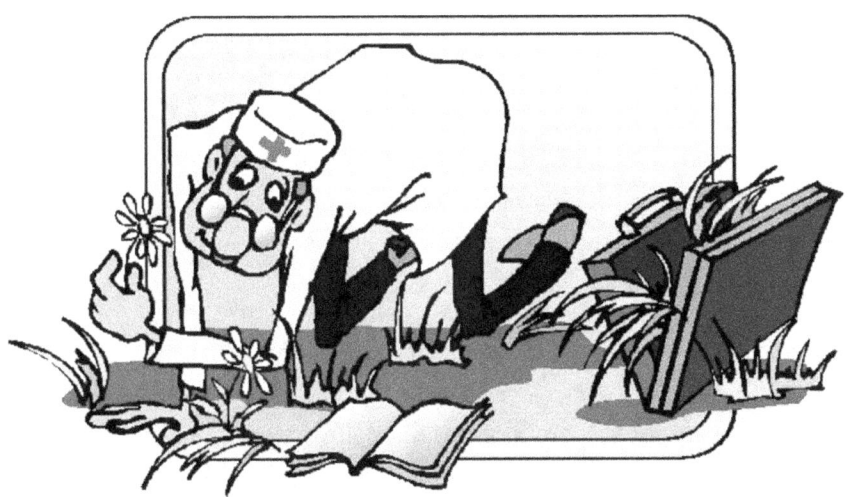

I had visions of growing all the herbs I needed to make all the natural medicine me and my family required. I had no interest in essential oils because that was not something I could grow and make myself.

When I became a massage therapist, essential oils became my main focus, because that is what we primarily use in our profession.

Although our main focus is on essential oils, we do however need to understand the broader picture of herbs and natural healing to truly understand and make better decisions when using essential oils in our profession. We need to understand what is in the products we are using on our clients and what is being absorbed into our bodies through our hands.

We read in magazines, televisions, radio programs the claims and miracles of herbs and essential oils. You cannot interchange herbs with essential oils. Remember that many of these stories are being told by writers and broadcasters not experienced in herbs and essentials oils. They are repeating the news or headliner of the day.

Natural healing is your best choice for chronic health conditions. Chemical medicines, surgery and other miracle of technology are best for acute conditions. Believe me, if I am in a car accident I want an emergency room not an herbalist or naturopath.

Anything that goes into or on your body that is not a product of a plant the body treats as a toxin. The liver and kidney processes these toxins. As long as the liver is functioning properly and is not overwhelmed with these toxins the body does not suffer damages.

Every day we are hearing of tragic results of overuse or side effects of chemical medicines. You know that warning label on Acetaminophen that says do not take with alcohol. I have a client whose wife did died from kidney failure after a cruise where she was drinking and taking Acetaminophen. I know someone whose pancreas was destroyed from too many antibiotics.

Name a few incidents you have heard of that are either side effects or injury from chemical drugs.

Because herbs are plants, there is not as great a threat of liver and chemical damage.

Herbs however, can be harmful. Overuse of Comfrey and Kava Kava can cause liver damage. Overuse of Ephedra can cause heart problems. Essential oils can be very dangerous when not used properly.

Essential Oils and herbal medicine are natural compliments to massage therapy. There are many passages using herbs or oil as a treatment for healing in all ancient manuscripts including the Bible.

Herbs come in many forms. Burning incense was used to cleanse the air, promote meditation at temples, and effect mood. Today we would use an atomizer or a room spray.

The most common treatment was to drink the herbs as a tea throughout the day and night. Herbs were made into tinctures or extracts, soaking them in alcohol or wine. Infusing herbs into oils with the addition of beeswax was used as a topical ointment to treat wounds or to massage into the skin as a treatment for muscles aches and pains. Herbal extracts can be added to nut butters to make suppositories. Herbs are effective in baths.

Essential oils are distilled parts of the plants that are inhaled or massaged into the skin. Some essential oils can be taken internally with caution.

Essential oil's constituents or properties only include those that are in the oil of the plant. There are many more constituents or properties remaining. Take an example, peppermint. The major properties of peppermint essential oil are, menthol, menthone, menthofurane, cineol, pulegone, menthyl acetae.

Left behind are Phenolic acids including rosmarinic acid, and flavonoids and tannins.

Essential oils do not mix with water. An herbal tincture or extract would work better in a mouthwash or other preparations requiring water.

As I learned more and more about herbs I discovered nutrition is even more important than herbal medicine. Herbs that are eaten as a food are called potherbs. In our grandmother's day that would be Polk Salad, dandelion greens, and other greens Today in natural healing many fruits and vegetables are juiced or blended as a healing remedy. So I suppose those fruits and vegetables that are juiced or blended for therapeutic benefits would be considered potherbs.

Then there is homeopathic, and Bach Flower Remedies and many other modalities.

Different methods of extracting herbs will extract different chemical properties of the herb. Some herbalists do not consider essential oils a true part of herbal medicine. They do not consider herbal medicines that extract only the "active chemical" that has been isolated as true herbal medicine. Their view is that all parts of the herbs work in synergy to create harmony in the body.

Herbs can be perfectly safe eaten, taken as a tincture or pill, or used in a bath but be quite dangerous as an essential oil.

Fresh or dried herbs are in one category while essential oils are a different category. We will start out discussing herbs.

Herbs can be used to treat the symptoms or treat the cause.

2 Methods of Extracting Herbs

Choosing which method to extract the healing properties of any given herb will depend on if the "active ingredient" is water soluble or alcohol soluble. Water soluble herbs can be taken as a tea. If the "active ingredient" is alcohol soluble it will be more therapeutic taken as a tincture. There are herbs that can be effective that are soaked in oil or glycerin. Today's newest technology extracts herbs by carbon dioxide, called super critical CO_2 promises to be the most exact and best form of extraction.

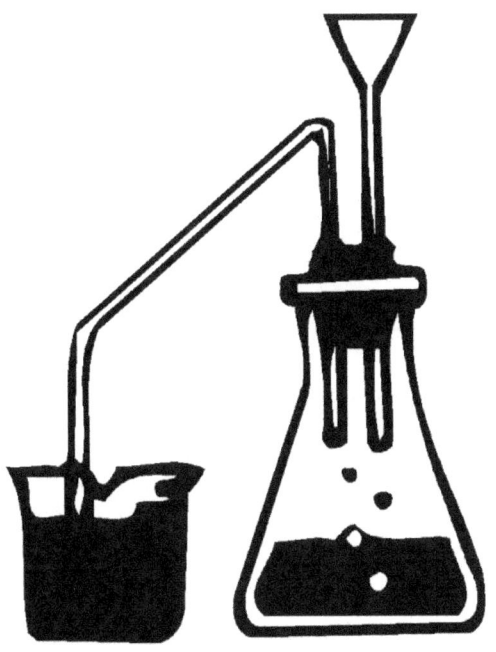

The Folk Method

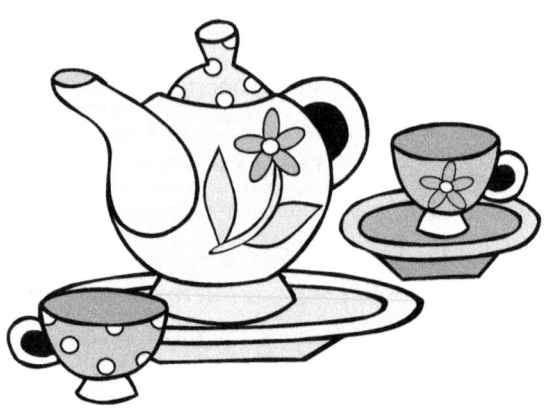

Herbal Tea
Hot Infusion for
leaves, flowers,
and green stems
1 cup boiling
water
1 teaspoon of
dried herb
or
3 teaspoons of
fresh herb
Steep 10-15
minutes

For centuries herbs (fresh or dried) were drank as teas. This is the simplest method and sometimes the most effective. Teas are drunk all through the day and night. Typically 1 cup three times a day. These teas can be used as a compress or as a poultice or poured into a bath. They can also be used as douches or enemas, make sure the tea is cooled to room temperature before use. They are made fresh each day as they will spoil.

Sometimes just the ritual of taking the time to stop and make a cup of tea or coffee would be part of the relaxing effect. Everyone knows that coffee is a stimulant, but how many people relax with a cup of coffee?

Leaves, flowers, and green stems and some seeds of the plants are used. If the herb is fresh it must be chopped in to tiny pieces. If the herb is dried it is crushed either with a mortar and pestle (old fashion method) or today's method would be a food or coffee grinder.

Hot Infusion

A glass or china teapot is first warmed with hot water, 1 teaspoon of dried herb or 3 teaspoons of fresh is added to the tea pot and 1 cup of boiling water per 1 cup of tea. The teapot is then covered with a lid and is allowed to steep for 10-15 minutes.

Cold Infusion

Cold infusions are used for herbs that are sensitive to heat and will lose their effectiveness. In this case, the herbs and water or milk are placed in a container with a tight fitting lid and allowed to sit for 6-12 hours. Do not use milk if the individual is allergic to milk.

Decoctions

When parts of the herb that is used is hard and woody such as the roots, rhizomes, bark, hard seeds, nuts, the mixture is brought to a boil and simmered for 10-15 minutes.

Of course there are always exceptions to the rules. Some roots contain volatile oils which would be destroyed by boiling. These herbs are finely powdered and infused with a tight fitting lid. Ginger, Saw Palmetto, and Turmeric come to mind.

If a herbal formula calls for both the leaves and flowers or a plant and the roots of another how do you think you would prepare it?

Decoctions
When parts of the herb that is used is hard and woody such as the roots, rhizomes, bark, hard seeds, nuts, the mixture is brought is a boil and simmered for 10-15 minutes

Mints

With all the exotic and foreign herbs to choose from, why begin with mints? Why not an herb that is new and exciting?

Mints are readily available, affordable and can be easily be grown at home. Their effectiveness has been proven in the marketplace and their effects are one of the few herbs that can be immediately demonstrated in the class room.

Herbs are divided into Genus, and then further defined into species. While an herb may be in the same Genus, the specific species may have different properties. The difference between Mentha piperita (Peppermint) and Mentha spicata (Spearmint) is easily demonstrated in class.

Mints are well known in the kitchen and deserve a healthy respect in your herbal remedy kit.

Project supplies needed:
Peppermint plant, dried Peppermint for tea or tea bag, bottle of essential oil of Peppermint, Spearmint plant, dried Spearmint for tea or tea bag, and essential oil of Spearmint.

Prepare a cup of Peppermint tea and a cup of Spearmint tea.

Mints are divided into 3 groups, cooking, healing, and decoration. All mints are refreshing and cooling. All mints have square stems. Most of them are perennials, and if not killed by a hard freeze or lack of water are very invasive and will spread by their roots. Control mint spreading in your garden by planting in pots or in a bottomless container at least 10 " deep. Different mints will interbreed. Keep the flowers pinched off and different mint plants as far away from each other as you can. When you purchase mints at the nursery, rub the leaves to check the aroma.

Mints originally came from Europe and Asia. Mint naturalized in

North America by the immigrants settling the country. Most mints are hardy to zone 5. It will grow in sun or shade with plenty of water. If you live in the southwest, like Texas, I can tell you from experience, spearmint will grow in full sun if given plenty of water. Peppermint is better grown in the shade.

Do not buy mint seeds. The only way to get the mint you really want is to propagate from cuttings or layering.

Peppermint: *Mentha piperita*

The most well know mint is Peppermint. This is the mint used medically and in most of your candies, breath mints and treats. Peppermint tea is a well known remedy for indigestion, cramps and headaches. The oil of peppermint is also well known as a remedy for toothaches and muscle soreness. Peppermint is the herb you would use with chocolate, coffee and candies.

The menthol in Peppermint is well known as a digestive aid. Everyone has inhaled menthol for respiratory problems. Menthol is the main ingredient in Vicks Rub. The vapors from Vicks Rub or other ointments containing menthol rubbed on the neck and chest help relieve a stuffy nose.

Peppermint grows closer to the ground, has smaller leaves than spearmint and is purple underneath its leaves and has purple stems. It requires more shade and more water than Spearmint.

Peppermint Tea

1 cup of boiling water
1 teaspoon dried Peppermint leaves or Peppermint tea bag, or 6-8 fresh leaves

Pour boiling water over the Peppermint, steep for 10 minutes. Strain

Take a sip. Pucker up and suck air through your lips. Notice the cool effect from the menthol in the Peppermint tea.

Touch the Peppermint plant. Rub the leaves between your fingers and then smell the leaves.

Sniff the bottle of essential oil of Peppermint.

Just take notice of the difference in fresh, cooked and distilled.

A cup of warm Peppermint tea will thin mucus and loosen phlegm and help relieve a stuffy nose. Peppermint tea is good as a digestive aid.

Peppermint for Headaches

Peppermint Headache Compress, good for sinus or tension headache

Add ice cubes to prepared peppermint tea. Wet washcloth in cold tea and apply to forehead.

Peppermint Tea Foot Soak

Pour 1 quart of boiling water over a handful for Peppermint leaves and let steep for 5 minutes. Use warm in the winter to stimulate circulation for colds and the flu. Add ice to make a soak for hot tired feet.

Peppermint for Itchy Eyes

Soak Peppermint tea bags in hot water for 30 minutes. Cool and place on eyes.

Cautions: Do not give to children under 3 Peppermint, do not use Peppermint if you have a Hiatal hernia or heartburn.

Spearmint and other mints

Spearmint: Mentha: spicata, or viridis
Sample the spearmint tea that was made. Now take a sip of cold
spearmint water.

Touch the Spearmint plant. Rub the leaves between your fingers and
then smell the plant.

Even though the Spearmint is cool and refreshing, notice there is no
menthol.

Spearmint, fruity mints and curly mints contain no menthol and are
generally used for cooking. Spearmint can be used instead of
Peppermint on children for inflammation and as an antiseptic.

Spearmint is what you would use to make a mint cucumber sauce or
use with lamb. Spearmint is the mint for Greek, Arabic, North
African, Indian and Middle Eastern dishes. Spearmint is the mint for
Mint Juleps, Mojitos, and other drinks.

Mint Juleps, Mojitios and Wriggly Spearmint gum! No wonder the
16 century herbalist wrote, "The smell rejoiceth the heart of man ".
And, I might add, it is the mint for lovers.

The aroma of Spearmint opens and releases emotional blocks and
brings about a feeling of well being and balance.

Spearmint is cooling and refreshing in the summer heat. Just
smelling the aroma seems to help cool you off.

Spearmint will grow in full sun even in Texas and get maybe 2 feet
tall. I have seen some varieties given more shade and more water get
3-4 feet tall. Giving the spearmint a little shade and more water will
give you bigger leaves. Cut it often to keep it shorter and keep it
from looking weedy and scraggly. Keeping it cut back will force the
stems to branch out and make the plants look lush and healthy, and

of course give you more leaves.

Spearmint is hardy to zone 5. It is a kind of a dark lime green, which is why I suppose it goes so well with limes and lemons. It has rough, jagged pointed leaves that grow up a square stem. The younger the stem the closer together the leaves will be. If you let your spearmint go too long without cutting it back, the leaves will grow further and further apart. If you can't drink that many Mojitios or mint tea or lemonade tie it up in little bundles and hang them around the house or on the porch for that little bit of fragrant cottage ambience. Or, of course, you might also be accused of being a witch.

Spearmint is invasive and will take over your garden. If you don't' absolutely love spearmint and think the more the better either grow it in a pot, or put a barrier of some sort around it at least 10" deep. It will grow through mulch and rocks.

Using spearmint in any of your bath or body products will be restorative and stimulating, according to Jeanne Rose, who also adds that spearmint feels good and strengthens the nerves and muscles. She also includes mint as one the 6 best herbs for cosmetics. Rose, Thyme, Comfrey, Mint, Lavender and Rosemary. Jeanne Rose's Herbal Body Book

Simple ways to use Spearmint:.

Bruise 1 cup of mint leaves, add to a half gallon pitcher (2 qt.), fill with water and refrigerate. After it is chilled, strain and serve over ice. You could also use this to rinse off your face or your body to cool off.

Add a sprig to your lemonade or ice tea.

Applemint, Pineapple Mint, and the other fruity mints are mostly used for garnishing drinks and flavoring things like cottage cheese.

LEMON BALM
Melissa officinalis

Lemon Balm or Melissa is referred to as the gladdening herb. It is often combined with hops and valerian to help with sleep and anxiety.

Lemon Balm is the mildest tranquilizer to calm anxiety and stress, safe even for children. It gently relaxes the digestive muscles and has been used for centuries to relieve colic and digestion problems.

Lemon Balm is for any kind of nervous tension and stress. It is soothing for coughs and colds and PMS. Although it can be soothing to irritated skin, the essential oil must be used in very small dilution because it can also cause skin irritation. It has antihistamine properties that will help with insect stings and helps heals wounds.

The extract of Lemon Balm is being used to decrease agitation in Alzheimer's patients and helps increase their memory.

Studies show Lemon Balm lip ointment applied 3-4 times a day shortens and lessen the severity of herpes outbreaks.

Lemon Balm may interfere with thyroid hormones.

See page 80 for formula for Lemon Balm lip ointment

3 Herbal Recipes

Spearmint

The Mojito Cocktail

Pronounced Mo-hee-toe
The Mojito is basically a limeade with rum and mint. The original Mojito was made with a particular mint from Cuba called Mojito. The word Mojito comes from the African word "mojo", meaning to cast a spell. The Mojito mint does not have the distinctive spearmint flavor. It has a very mild spearmint flavor and tastes a little more herby or earthy. I myself prefer spearmint to the Mojito mint.

Because trade with Cuba is prohibited, the Mojito mint has not been available in the states. In 2006 the Mojito mint came to the United States through Canada making the authentic Mojito Cocktail available to all. The Mojito cocktail was Eernest Hemingway's favorite drink and became a celebrity today when ordered by James Bond in the film, "Die Another Day."

EVER REGION CALLS ITS RECIPE THE AUTHENTIC ONE. IF YOU GO TO COZMUEL THEIR BARTENDERS CLAIM THEIR RECIPE IS THE REAL THING. I HAVE HAD A MOJITO AT A MIAMI FLORIDA AIRPORT. THE BARTENDER CLAIMED HIS FATHER CAME FROM CUBA AND BROUGHT THE ORIGINAL RECIPE. I OFFER YOU SEVERAL VARIANCES

Mojito Cocktail Recipe

4 fresh Mojito mint leaves
2 ounces lime juice, fresh is better, bottled if that is all you have, or a combination of both
1 teaspoon powdered sugar
2 ounces white rum
2 ounces club soda

Lime wedge and mint sprig for garnish

In a tall class smash (muddle) together the mint leaves, the lime juice and the powdered sugar with a muddler, spoon or whatever you can find. Add ice and rum and stir. Then add the club soda and garnish with a wedge of lime and a sprig of mint. Do not try to add the rum when you are smashing the lime, mint and sugar together. Sugar does not dissolve well in alcohol. That is why you add the rum afterwards.

Cozmel Mojito

Springs of spearmint
1/3 cup lime juice
1/3 cup sugar syrup
2 oz rum
Water, ice, lime slices and spearmint leaves for garnish

The bartender here used sugar syrup. Sugar syrup is made by heating equal amounts of water and sugar together until the sugar dissolves completely. The sugar syrup is then refrigerated until ready to use.

Use an 8 oz glass or larger.
Muddle Spearmint leaves in 1/3 cup of lime juice.
Stir in 1/3 cup of sugar syrup.
Stir in 2 oz. rum
Top off with water and ice.

Tzatzito Sauce

1 onion chopped fine
1 cucumber
1 cup Greek yogurt
1 T lemon juice
1-2 T chopped Jalapenos
7-10 spearmint leaves
Garlic clove
Salt to taste

Peel and chop cucumber, place inside a colander and place something heavy on top to drain juice from cucumbers.
Blend all ingredients in a food processor except salt. Taste and then add salt to taste.

Basil

Dogwood Gardens Basil Pesto
3 cups of fresh basil
1 oz of fresh garlic(whole bulb of cloves)
½ cup walnuts
½ cup grated parmesan cheese
3 T Romano cheese (optional)
2/3 cup of olive oil
1 T lemon juice
Pinch of salt

Process Basil, garlic, and olive oil in food processor. Add cheese and nuts, lemon juice and salt. Blend

Serving suggestion:
While tortellini is still hot mix in pesto, just enough to coat. Add fresh or sundried tomatoes. Refrigerate.

Scoop out the inside of cherry tomatoes and fill with pesto

Split French bread, spread with pesto, sliced tomatoes, feta cheese or other cheese and broil.

Another delicious way to enjoy Basil: Combine sliced cherry tomatoes and chopped basil. Add pressed garlic and cover half way with olive oil. Add a little salt. Refrigerate to mingle flavors and serve.

Mexican Marigold Vinegar:

Harvest the leaves and wash. Lay the leaves out to dry. Fill a quart jar with the fresh leaves. Crush the leaves. Bring a quart of vinegar almost to a boil and pour over the leaves. If using a metal cap to cover your jar, first place wax paper or plastic wrap between your jar and the lid. The vinegar will rust the metal lid. Shake the jar 2 x a day for a month. Strain into another clean container. Place a few leaves in for identification.

A great way to recycle those Starbucks Frappicino bottles is to use them for your herbal vinegars. You will need to place a piece of plastic wrap or waxed paper between the lid and the bottle to prevent the lid from rusting.

Cucumber and Onion Salad:

¼ cup of Mexican Marigold Mint Vinegar
¼ cup of sugar or honey.

Mix the vinegar and sweetener together in a shallow container, such as a pie dish. Add sliced cucumbers and onions. Coat the cucumbers and onions. Cover with plastic wrap and place in the refrigerator for 30 minutes to an hour before serving.

Instead of Poppy Seed Dressing, substitute the vinegar for MMM Vinegar and add chopped MMM leaves.

¾ cup sugar, or honey, or agave
1/3 cup of MMM vinegar
1 teaspoon salt
½ cup of your choice of oil
¼ cup of chopped MMM leaves

Combine the sugar, vinegar and salt. Use a blender to gradually add in the oil and emulsify. Store in the refrigerator until you are ready to use.

This is good over fruit salads, spinach salads, and avocados.

HERBAL VINEGARS

Herbal Vinegars are basically all made the same. Once made they can be used as a facial tonic, vinegar pie, a base for salad dressings, fruit salads dressings, marinades, and vinaigrettes.

You can use apple cider vinegar, champagne vinegar, wine vinegar, the choice is yours.

Although I use natural unpasteurized vinegar in my kitchen the only time I have had herbal vinegars mold is when I used all natural, unpasteurized vinegar. Use with your discretion.

Wash herbs before using. Let the herbs dry. Too much water left on your herbs will dilute the acidity of the vinegar. The acidity of the vinegar is what preserves the mixture.

Herbal Vinegar

Fill quart jar with bruised herb leaves (about 3 cups), bulb of garlic(optional). Fill jar with heated vinegar. Not boiling just to the boiling point. Cover jar with lid and shake 2 times a day for 10 days to 2 weeks. Strain vinegar into decorative jar and add fresh herb leaves for decoration and identification. Purple Basil makes a beautiful pink vinegar.

Use to make an vinaigrette.
Oil, Vinegar, water, vegetable juice, salt, pepper, other herbs to taste.

Hot Vinaigrette:
Fry 6 slices of bacon. Remove bacon. Add 2 T sugar, 2 T herbal vinegar, powdered garlic. Bacon should have enough salt that salt is not needed but taste and add salt if necessary. Crumble bacon over salad.

Rosemary Punch

1 tablespoon of dried Rosemary or a sprig of fresh
1 tablespoon of dried Lemon Balm or a sprig of fresh
1 large can of pineapple juice
1 liter of Gingerale
½ cup of lemon juice
1 ½ quarts of water
Optional: sliced strawberries and sliced lemon for garnish.

Bring water to a boil. Pour over crushed herbs. Cover and steep until cool. Strain. Add herb tea to the other ingredients. Float strawberries and lemon slices in punch.

Homemade Ginger Ale #1

1 inch fresh Ginger root, peeled grated, or chopped
¾ cup sugar
1/8 teaspoon yeast
Water

Grate 1 inch of fresh Ginger root, combine in a sauce pan with 1 cup of water, and ¾ cup of sugar. Cook over medium heat until the sugar is dissolved. Remove from heat, cover and steep for 1 hour. Strain this syrup and refrigerate for 1 hour. Pour into a 1 litre or 1 qt. container with a tight fitting lid. Add 1/8 teaspoon of active dry yeast, 6 cups of water, and 2 tablespoons of fresh lemon juice. Shake well, leave at room temperature for 2 days. (if using plastic bottles, the bottle will become hard when you try to squeeze them) and then refrigerate and use within 10 days. Add sparkling water or club soda to taste.

Homemade Ginger Ale #2

¾ cup of Ginger root peeled and finely chopped or grated
½ cup lime juice
¼-1/2 cup of sugar
2 teaspoons of salt
2 quarts of water
¼ cup of whey

Place all ingredients into a 2 quart container with a tight fitting lid. Leave at room temperature 2-3 days. If using plastic bottles, the bottle will become hard when you try to squeeze them. Refrigerate. Will keep several months.
Whey: Strain 1 quart of yogurt (not Greek yogurt) that has no fillers or sweeteners, into a strainer covered with cheesecloth, leave for 12-24 hours. The liquid coming out will be whey. The yogurt will now be Greek Yogurt.

Quick Homemade Ginger Ale

1 cup peeled, finely chopped or grated Ginger root
2 cups water
1 cup of sugar and 1 cup of water
Club soda, lime juice

Add 1 cup of the grated Ginger to 2 cups of boiling water. Reduce heat and simmer the Ginger for 5 minutes. Remove from heat and steep for 20 minutes. Strain.
Make a simple syrup dissolving the 1 cup of sugar into the 1 cup boiling water.

For each glass of Ginger Ale, mix ½ cup of Ginger water with 1/3 cup of simple syrup and ½ cup of club soda. Add a squeeze of lime juice.

Natural Ginger Ale

1 teaspoon of fresh grated Ginger or ½ teaspoon of powdered ginger
Optional : sprig of lemon balm or other lemon scented herb
3 cups of water
1 cup of carbonated water
Lime or lemon juice
Sweetener of choice

Combine Ginger and plain water in a saucepan and bring to a boil. If using sugar, add sugar now (1/2 – 1cup of sugar) Simmer for 5 minutes. Remove from heat (add lemon scented herb) and steep for 20 minutes. Strain and refrigerate. Add carbonated water and ¼ cup - 1/2 cup of lemon or lime juice.

Try using your Soda Stream. Cook equal amounts of the grated Ginger, Sugar, and Water to make a syrup. Add a little of the syrup to your Soda Stream.

Herbal Honey

Scald glass jars. Add 2-5 tablespoons of chopped fresh herbs to 1 pint (2 cups) of honey. Place in sunny location for 5-10 days, strain and rebottle.

Fruit Dip:
Add 2-3 tablespoons of herbal honey to 1 cup of sour cream or yogurt

Herb Honey Butter
Add ½ cup of herb honey to 1 cup of butter
Use to glaze chicken or season vegetables

Use in the center of cookies

4 Tinctures, Extracts and Oils

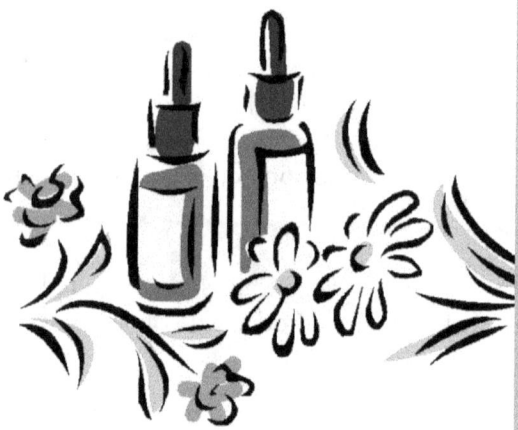

Homemade Tinctures

4 oz. of dried herb to 1 pint of 60 – 80 proof alcohol

Or

8 oz of fresh herb To 1 pint of 60 – 80 proof alcohol

Shake 2 x a day, for 6 weeks, strain and store in dark bottle.

Tinctures are made with alcohol or vinegar. Sometimes they are mistakenly called extracts. Tinctures are more concentrated than teas so you use less, and the alcohol acts as a preservative. Tinctures stored in a cool dark place may have a shelf life up to 1-2 years.

Commercially made tinctures have an exact ratio of alcohol to herb varying with each herb and different standards. Homemade tinctures are made by chopping or grinding 4 oz of dried herb or 8 oz fresh herb and adding 1 pint of 60-80 proof Vodka, to a container with a tight fitting lid. Most people will use canning jars. Because 60 or 80 proof Vodka has both alcohol and water, properties that are water soluble and alcohol soluble are extracted from the herb. Other alcohols can be used but Vodka is the standard. Wine can be used with some herbs such as elderberry wine. This mixture is kept in a warm place for 6 weeks and shook twice a day. The first 2 weeks check this mixture to make sure the Vodka completely covers the herbs, add more Vodka if necessary. It is then strained and poured into dark colored bottle with a tight fitting lid.

Since the strength of a homemade tincture will vary these are used when the dosage is not critical.

Fresh leaves and flowers are considered more effective than dried root tinctures. The whole top of the plant is juiced and then alcohol is added as a preservative. Juice the plant, measure and then add 1/3 as much alcohol. Let set for 7 days and filter. Store in a dark bottle.

Tinctures can be taken straight, added to water or other liquids, used to make ointments, salves, suppositories and lozenges.

Important tinctures to have on hand would be Echinacea for wounds, infections, colds and the flu. A tincture of Elderberries would go along with Echinacea for colds and flu if you did not want the sugar or honey in the Elderberry syrups.

A tincture of Hops would be valuable to have on hand for insomnia and inflammation.

A tincture of Sage mixes well with water as a mouthwash for dental problems and fresh breath.

Fluid or Liquid Extracts

These are commercially made products with specific weight and measurements and technical equipment and skills. These are made with alcohol and glycerin. You can get precise doses and they can be standardized to have a certain amount of the active ingredient.

Syrups

Syrup can be as easy as adding 1 part tincture to 3 parts of a simple syrup mixture and store in the refrigerator.

Simple Syrup

To 1 pint of water add 2 ½ pounds of sugar. Stir to dissolve, bring to a boil and remove from heat.

Another method would be to add ¾ pounds of sugar to 1 pint of tincture and stir on low heat until the sugar is dissolved.

Herbal Honey Syrup:[1]

Add (1/4 cup) of dried herb or ½ cup of fresh herb to 1 quart (4 cups) of water. Boil down and reduce to 1 pint (2 cups)

Strain and add 2-4 tablespoons of honey. Store in the refrigerator for up to 1 month

Elderberry Syrup:

First make elderberry juice by simmering 1 gallon of ripe elderberries with ½ cup of water for 1 hr. Optional: add ½ ounce of ginger root and 18 whole cloves.
Strain and bottle when cool, store in the refrigerator.
Pour 4 oz. into a glass, add hot water and honey to taste.

Elderberry Syrup 2
Elderberry syrup is basically elderberry jelly without the pectin.
Wash canning jars or bottles. Sterilize jars by boiling for 15 minutes or run through dishwasher on the hot cycle.
Soak lids and bands in hot water.

Add enough water to cover bottom of pan and add elderberries. Crush elderberries and simmer for 15 minutes. Pour juice and berries and strain through cheesecloth.

---

[1] Growing and Using the Healing Herbs by Gaea and Shandor Weiss

Measure 1 cup of sugar per 1 cup of juice.
Measure 3 tablespoons of lemon juice per 1 cup of juice.

Bring the elderberry juice to a boil. Add the sugar and the lemon juice. Bring to a full rolling boil and stir for 1 minute. Remove from heat and skim off foam. Fill jars immediately. Wash off top of jars and cover with lids and bands. Bathe in a water bath process for 15 minutes. Take 1 tablespoon 4 times per day.

Dried Elderberries:

½ cup of dried Elderberries
5 cloves
12 star anise (see note below)
2 cinnamon sticks
Options: add licorice root or ginger. If you do not have the cloves, cinnamon, or star anise, make the syrup without them.
2 cups of water
1 cup of honey

Combine the elderberries, star anise, cinnamon sticks, and cloves. Bring to boil and simmer for 30-45 minutes or until reduced to ½. Strain. Cool and then stir in honey. Place in jar and refrigerate for a couple of weeks. Freeze in small containers for longer storage.

Take 1 tablespoon at the first sign Use as a cough syrup.
As a cough syrup: adults, take 1 tablespoon every hour for cough.
Children: ½ to 1 teaspoon ever 2-3 hours.
According to an 2011 article in Alternative Medicine Studies, Star Anise is the primary source of shikimic acid, the precursor to oseltamivir, the anti viral medication known as Tamiflu.

Juicing
Fruits and Vegetables that are juiced or blended.

Potherbs
Usually greens of some sort that are cooked and eaten.

Suppositories

Suppositories are made with cocoa butter or other nut butter and mixed with a finely powdered herb or they can be made with a mixture of gelatin, glycerin and an herbal tincture or decoction.

Ointments and Salves

An ointment or salve begins with an herbal oil. The herbal oil is then thickened with beeswax. 1 oz. of beeswax per 8 oz. of herbal oil. There are countless recipes and methods.

Herbal oils are as simple as soaking the dried herb in oil. Macerate 4 tablespoons of dried herb or ½ cup of fresh herb with 2 cups of vegetable oil, let sit in a dark place for 3 days and then strain and bottle. I always add Vitamin E to help preserve it.

These oils will go rancid and should be stored in the refrigerator.

Herbal Oil 2:

Heat the herbs and oil in a pot for 1 hour not letting the oil get over 2oo°F.

To me it is easier to pour the herbs and oils into a casserole dish, place in the oven and set the oven for 1-2 hours. Strain and bottle. I normally pour the herbal oil back into the vegetable oil bottle I used and store in the refrigerator. I pour a small amount into a medicine bottle for everyday use.

If your crockpot's lowest setting is below 200°F you could use that.

The herbal oils most used in massage would be Arnica and St. John's Wort. Wort by the way means herb.

Liniments

Liniments are made with rubbing alcohol and sometimes vinegar. These can be made from an herbal tincture or made with essential oils. They can be used to stimulate muscles and ligaments or used to relax muscles and ligaments. They are meant to go through the skin and never taken internally.

Do you remember the home remedy of soaking raisins in gin for arthritis? Juniper berries are used in gin as a flavor ingredient. Juniper berries are a Native American remedy for arthritis.

Allopathic or chemical medicines normally have only one benefit. Herbs can have many different benefits and sometimes seem opposite to each other. Peppermint and Lavender can be both relaxing and stimulating.

When you see a list of herbs to treat certain conditions you must consider what is causing the symptoms. Herbal medicine is more effective in some forms than others.

When you inhale Peppermint it does help with sinus congestion. But you can smell it all day long and is not going to help your pain. It could help certain headaches when inhaled. But for most headaches and muscle pain, it has to be massaged into the muscle. In this case an essential oil of Peppermint would be more effective. Drinking a cup of Peppermint tea, or sucking on a Peppermint candy would work better for an upset stomach.

Ginger is more effective taken eternally for nausea that being rubbed on as an essential oil.

For me menstrual cramps or intestinal cramps are better relieved taking Black Cohosh internally than having an essential oil rubbed onto my belly.
Recommended essential oils for massaging on the cramping area would be Basil, Tarragon and Clary Sage. [2]

---

[2] Natural Home Health Care Using Essential Oils by Daniel Penoel and Rose-Marie Penoel

You as a massage therapist may have a massage technique to relieve cramps and the essential oil would be a compliment to your massage technique.
Does anyone here have a special technique for menstrual cramps?

After the birth of my son I had a headache that lasted 20 years. Sometimes the headaches were so bad they put me to bed, other times they were just barely there. I tried all the herbal remedies for headaches, relaxation, and sinus congestion.

I took Ephedra the natural relief for sinus congestion and asthma. They did not help my headaches but I did have incredible energy and lost 10 pounds. By the way, Ephedra is not safe for those with high blood pressure. When Ephedra was the big diet craze it was because of a synthesized version of the main chemical which was dangerous for those with high blood pressure and could also cause high blood pressure. Because of misuse Ephedra has been taken off the market.

I searched for Umeboshi a Japanese plum pickled in salt, because they were suppose to be the ultimate thing to restore me to an alkaline ph. Another natural cure for headaches.

It wasn't until I discovered how to treat myself with trigger point therapy that I relieved my headaches.

St John's Wort is the main herb for sciatica or nerve pain. It is not an essential oil but is available as pills, tinctures, or as an infused oil. From my experience, decompression exercises and Trigger Point Treatments will treat the cause. St. John's Wort will soothe the irritated nerves.

From the American Indians to the Orient, from the deepest parts of Africa to the lands of the Bible God has given mankind healing herbs. Different parts of the world will have herbs that are traditionally used to treat certain complaints. Herbalists are going to use herbs that they are familiar with or according to what grows in their country. I have many, many books on herbs. I have never read of Basil being used for the heart or chest pain. Local Mexican workers came to my farm wanting Basil when one of them was having chest pains. Another worker made a tea from the leaves of the mesquite tree to treat pink eye. Every herb book I have ever read uses eyebright with no mention of the mesquite tree.

For centuries, herbal healing has relied on tradition and by observation. Now that herbs and essential oils are becoming main stream much clinical research is being done.

5 Herbs for the Bath

The easiest way to add herbs to your bath is to fill a cloth bag or sock with ½ to 1 cup of dried herbs and either hang from the tub faucet or allow the bag to float in the tub, but not the most effective. The most effective way to add herbs to your bath is to first make a tea and then add that to your bath.

Heat 1 quart of water to the boiling point and pour over 1 cup of fresh herbs or ½ cup of dried herbs. Cover and let steep at least 20 minutes, strain and pour tea into your bath water.

If using roots, tree bark or other woody parts boil the roots 2-5 minutes and then steep for 10-15 minutes.

The exception is fresh Ginger root, which you would steep in hot water for 20 minutes.

Herbal baths will not have the strong fragrance you may be accustomed to as when using essential oils or synthetic bath products.

 The Lord has provided herbs all over the world for all environmental conditions. The list of healing herbs are endless. Many have been forgotten, while others are being rediscovered.

Many herbs have multiple uses that seem to contradict each other. Herbs appear to have an inner knowledge to know which of its properties are needed by the body. Herbs such as Lavender can be both relaxing and stimulating. Ginger can raise or lower blood pressure.

This is a partial list. There are no plants on earth that someone is not allergic to. Use these herbs with discretion.

Beauty Herbs:

Ninon de L' Enclos, a French beauty who remained lovely into her 70's attributed her beauty to the power of her "Magic Waters", an herbal mixture of Comfrey, Rosemary, Lavender and Thyme.

Comfrey contains allantoin. Many believe with continuous use Comfrey regenerates aging tissue. Comfrey's high mucilage content makes it moisturizing and soothing to dry or irritated skin.

Rosemary is an energizing herb.

Lavender is an astringent that reduces puffiness and stimulates the complexion.

Thyme acts as an antiseptic.

Adding roses to this mix will add beauty and fragrance which would be soothing emotionally and physically.

Bruises, Cuts and Swelling

Remember a cool bath is better for bruises and swellings. First make an herbal tea to add to your bath. Injured hands, wrist, feet or ankles can be soaked in cold water in a large dishpan. Soak no more than 15 minutes per hour. Adding Epsom salts or sea salts would enhance the therapeutic values.

After the swelling has gone down, alternating hot and cold water soaks will speed the healing process.

Warm or hot water is better for cuts and injuries that are not swollen. Warm or hot water will help draw out toxins and bring in fresh red blood to speed the healing process.

Enhance the healing process with these herbs:
Bay, Chamomile, Comfrey, Echinacea, Elder, Lavender, Marjoram, Mints, Mugwort, Oregano, Plantain, Thyme, Wintergreen Yarrow.

POISON IVY AND OTHER SKIN IRRITATIONS

Comfrey, Kelp, Mullein, Oats, Parsley, Sage, Stinging Nettles

If you are allergic to poison ivy grow Comfrey. The juice from the fresh leaf gives remarkable results.
Add 1 cup of vinegar or herbal to your bath.

Soothing herbs:
Soothing herbs are food and tonics for the nervous system. They help us cope with every day stress. They are healing to the mind and the body. Use these herbs to relax after a stressful day.

Calendula, Chamomile, Clary Sage, Comfrey, Elder Flowers, Jasmine flowers, Juniper berries, Lavender flowers, Lemon Balm, Mullein, Oats, Passion flowers, Pine Needles, Roses

Soothing Herbs that help you sleep:
Chamomile, Hops, Dill, Lavender flowers, Lemon Balm, Oats, Valerian, Yarrow, Mugwort (in the bath or use in a sleeping pillow do not consume)

Stimulating Herbs:

Stimulating herbs increase blood circulation, increase energy, and warms the body. Stimulating herbs open the pores and promote sweating. This is called detoxifying. Use these herbs when you are cold, or sick with the cold or flu.
Muscular activity creates lactic acids. Lactic acids causes muscular aches and pains and fatigue. Stimulating herbs helps detoxify these acids. Increased circulation renews your energy and spirit.
Stimulating herbs enhance the detoxifying effects of bath salts.

Basil, Bay, Cayenne, Cinnamon, Cloves, Eucalyptus, Fennel, Ginger, Juniper, Horseradish roots, Lavender flowers, Lemon verbena, Mints, Mugwort, Mustard, Nasturtium, Nutmeg, Oregano(this is safe as an herb not as an essential oil), Pepper, Pine needles, Roses, Rosemary,

Sage, Stinging nettles, Strawberry leaves, Tarragon, Thyme, Wintergreen, Yarrow.

Caution: Wear gloves when handling Sting Nettles. First make a tea and then strain for the bath.

Rejuvenating Herbs:

Rejuvenating herbs renew the body, mind and spirit. Use these herbs when you feel drained, strained, and all used up. Use these herbs when you need to start all over again. Rejuvenating herbs refresh your skin after a long winter or too much time in the sun.

Anise, Carnation, Chamomile, Citrus Peelings, Comfrey, Fennel, Jasmine flowers, Lavender flowers, Oats, Rosemary, Yarrow

Up-lifting herbs:
Use these up lifting herbs to help you through a time of loss and sorrow.

Citrus peelings, Lemon Verbena, Marjoram, Oregano, Rosemary

6 Bath Additives and Formulas

Apple Cider Vinegar:

No, you will not smell like a salad. Apple cider vinegar added to your bath water relaxes, soothes and removes itchy, scaly skin. Vinegar helps detoxify sore, achy muscles. Ad ½ - 1 cup of vinegar to your bath to restore your body's natural PH. Skin that is too acidic can cause bacterial infections. Skin that is too alkaline can cause flaky and scaly skin. Vinegar helps fight fungal infections.

Vinegar Facial Tonic: Use to restore skin's PH
2 cups of distilled water
¼ cup of apple cider vinegar
10 drops of essential oil

Epsom's salts (magnesium sulfate):
Detoxifies sore achy muscle. Use one half to one pound of salts to a tub of hot water (105-110ºF.) 20-30 minutes. Do not rinse off the salts.

Borax:
Sodium borate, is a mineral powder used as a water softener and adds light bubbles to a bath blend. This is the same borax found in the cleaning section of the grocery store.

Baking Soda:
Sodium bicarbonate, softens bath water. Soda is alkaline helps relieve itching of irritated skin. Use one pound per bath.

Oats:
Oatmeal can be ground into a fine powder, soothing to irritated skin. It can be bought as oat straw, or in the grocery store as the same

oatmeal you buy for breakfast. Oats help relieve itching caused by poison ivy and poison oak.

Milk or cream: Smoothes and whitens the skin.

Sulphur:
Sulphur is a blood cleanser and purifier. Add 3-6 tablespoons to a hot bath (105-110ºF) and soak for 10-20 minutes. Doctors recommend sulphur for chronic muscle pain, neuritis, autointoxication, gout and skin diseases.

Sea Salt:
Sea salt is dried from sea water and is healing to open sores and is stimulating, increasing circulation. Use 1-3 pounds of salt in water warm water (90-94ºF) 10-20 minutes for a therapeutic bath.

Use sea salts for foot baths, stimulating and detoxifying baths.

Honey:
Honey is considered a humectant, meaning it pulls moisture from the air. Honey softens and moisturizes dehydrated or flaky skin. Honey is a naturally antiseptic, is anti fungal and is an antibacterial agent. From ancient times honey has been used as a wound dressing.

BATH CRYSTALS AND BATH SALTS

Bath salts can be as simple as buying rock salt, kosher salt, sea salt or even table salt and adding essential oils to them. Salts are drying. Bath crystals made with baking soda and cornstarch will leave your skin silky smooth.

Use 3-4 tablespoons for an aromatic bath. Use 1-2 cups for a therapeutic bath.

1 part baking soda
1 part sea salt
10-30 drops of essential oil

1 part sea salt
1 part Epsom salts
1 part Kosher salt
½ t glycerin for every 3 cups
10-30 drops of essential oil

2 parts baking soda
1 part cornstarch
10-30 drops of essential oil

2 parts Epsom salts
1 part Borax
1 part baking soda
10-30 drops of essential oil

Layer sea salts with fresh citrus peelings, rosemary leaves or other fresh herbs in a large mouth jar and cover with lid and let set.

Add sea salt to cool water to simulate the therapeutics benefits of the ocean.

FOOT BATHS

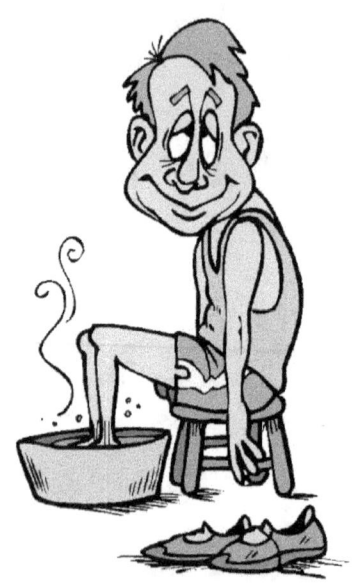

*Use warm water for a
relaxing foot bath
92-98°f
Soak 10-15 minutes*

*Use room temperature
water to refresh and
invigorate.
Soak 5 minutes*

Everyday muscular activity creates lactic acids. Gravity bring these fatigue causing acids to your feet. A salt water soak has a poultice like effect drawing fatigue acids out through the skin of your feet.

A warm water foot soak (92-98°f) is relaxing and will prepare you for a good night's sleep.

Water at room temperature is refreshing and invigorating and will prepare you for a night on the town.

Relaxing foot bath:
Prepare for a good night's sleep
1 cup of sea salt
4-6 quarts of warm water 92-98°f
5 drops of Lavender essential oils or other relaxing essential oils

Soak feet 15-20 minutes

Refreshing and Invigorating Foot Bath

Prepare for a night on the town.

2 cups of sea salt
1 gallon of water at room temperature
5 drops of essential oil of Peppermint or Rosemary or other stimulating essential oils.

Soak feet 5 minutes

Milk Baths

Cleopatra claimed milk baths and special herbs to be her beauty secrets. Milk can be added to the bath as instant milk powders, fresh milk, cream, buttermilk, or yogurt. Milk makes the skin feel smooth and soft as it whiten the skin. Buttermilk and yogurt contain lactic acid, said to kill bacteria. Add essential oils to milk or cream or try these formulas.

Use ½ cup per bath. Store in the refrigerator.

2 parts instant milk powder
1 part Epsom salts
10-30 drops essential oil

2 parts instant milk powder
1 part baking soda
1 part Epsom salts
10-30 drops of essential oil

2 cups instant milk powder
½ cup vegetable or nut oil
10-30 drops of essential oil

2 parts instant milk powder
1 part ground oatmeal
10-30 drops of essential oil

When combining large amounts of bath salts or crystals, mix a small amount of mixture with the essential oils and then add that mixture to the larger batch of bath salts or crytals.

Bath Oils

Bath oils are added to the bath to moisturize and scent the bath. 2 teaspoons of vegetable or nut oils from your kitchen can be used in the tub. Most of the oils float on top of the water, coating your skin when you step out of the tub. If you want an oil that mixes with the water, use castor oil. 10-30 drops of essential oil can be added to your oil of choice.
Safflower oil contains essential fatty acids to help damaged skin.
Grapeseed oil is light and non-greasy.
Apricot, avocado and sunflower oils are also good for the bath.

Oil does not moisturize the skin. Oil holds in the moisture that is already there. So, when you take a bath, soak in the tub for 10 minutes. This gives your skin a chance to soak up the water. Then you add the oil to trap in the moisture. When you add the oil first, you may be preventing the moisture from penetrating your skin. Spending more than 20 minutes in the tub will dry out your skin.

Adding bath oil to your bath tub can be dangerous. It will leave your tub slick. With the new synthetic tubs, oil is hard to clean off the tub. If you shower and do not take a bath to begin with you can still benefit from herbal oils.

After a shower or a bath leave the skin moist and apply the oil all over your body. Wrap yourself in an old gown or housecoat until the oil has been absorbed. You do not want to ruin your favorite gown with oil stains.

7 About Essential Oils

Essential Oils are distilled herbs or flowers. This is the concentrated essence of the plant. Citrus oils are pressed from the skin of the fruit, orange, grapefruit, lemon or lime. Jasmine is not an essential oil but an absolute. Absolutes use chemical extraction, so know your source and the chemical used during extraction before using therapeutically. Essential oils are also made from distilling tree resin such as Frankincense and Myrrh.

Aromatherapy uses these concentrated essences as an alternative therapy to promote the body's natural healing process to achieve balance and harmony. As essential oils evaporate they are inhaled, entering the body through the millions of cells that line the nasal passages effecting the body's psychological well being through the limbic system. Information from what we smell is sent to specific areas of the brain that influence memory, learning, basic emotions, hormonal balances and the flight or fight response. When essential oils are mixed with oils and lotions and massaged into the skin their tiny molecule structure allow them to penetrate the skin affecting the body physically. The fats that are used as carrier oils lie on the skin surface.

The Chinese were probably the first to discover the medical power of plants around 4500 B.C., but the Egyptians refined the art. All major civilizations and religions used essential oils.

The term "Aromatherapy" was termed in 1928 by the French chemist René Maurice Gatteforsse to describe the therapeutic action of essential oils.

Essential oils are very concentrated so they are used by drops. They normally are not taken orally but used instead by either inhalation are being diluted with lotions and massaged into the skin depending on the treatment required. You can buy a diffuser to diffuse the oil or use a cool mist humidifier. I personally don't like heat diffusion, but that is a matter of personal preference. Heat will destroy part of the medical benefits.

Everyone knows the benefits of using Eucalyptus and Peppermint for respiratory ailments and pain relief . A mixture of Eucalyptus and Peppermint can be rubbed on the temples or forehead for some type headaches. Basil can be used for some type headaches. Lavender is good for tension type headaches. Generally if over the counter pain relievers help your headaches these oils will work. If you have the type headache that do not respond to pain medication these essential oils will probably not work either.

Research by Dr. Dembar of the University of Cincinnati showed that inhaling Peppermint oil increased the mental accuracy of students by 28%. Rosemary is also good for memory.

Rose scented oils and Citrus oils are uplifting. Lavender is calming.

Nearly all essential oils have anti-bacterial qualities. Lemon oil is used in many European hospitals as an antiseptic instead of drugs. The main benefit of using essential oils are that bacteria and virus do not mutate to essential oils as they mutate to drugs.

Research now indicates that essential oils may be the drug of the future to aid in treating emotional and mental disorders. In 1989 it was discovered that the amygdala (a gland of the brain) plays a major role in storing and releasing emotional trauma. Only odor or fragrance stimulation has a profound effect in triggering a response with this gland.

Certain essential oils, do not cover up odors in your home but will

**actually break the odors down and eliminate the offending
odor. Synthetic oils cannot do this.**

Diffusing some oils in your home will help eliminate airborne
bacteria. Tea Tree oil is used for fungal infections.

We experience aromatherapy everyday of our lives. We smell bread
baking or charcoal and lighter fluid and we get hungry. A lady
wearing perfume passing by may make us feel pleasant or give us a
headache. A skunk or a rotting dead animal may make us feel
nauseated. Real Estate agents may burn a candle with the scent of
chocolate chips cookies to give the property a feeling of home.
Detailers give a used car that final touch with a new car scent.

Aromas can bring back memories. As a young wife back in the
seventies a friend brought over fresh baked yeast bread. I instantly
did not like the smell of the bread. I now realize it was because I
spent 3 years in Buckner Baptist Children's Home where they had
their own bakery. Each day the smell of yeast bread baking circulated
around the entire campus. At the time I did not know why I disliked
the smell of the bread but it still effected me. I now love yeast
bread.

Have you heard the saying, Pine- Sol clean?

Back in my day, the only cleaning products were Pine- Sol and Lysol.

When I smell the original Lysol scent I think of Buckner Baptist
Children's Home. We used Lysol there. When I smell Pine- Sol, I
think of home because that is what my mother cleaned with.

My first husband was injured in Viet Nam and spent 17 months in
the hospital at Fort Sam Houston. Later he could not enter a hospital
to visit family or friends because the scent of a hospital made him
sick. He later died in a construction accident.

Essential oils can affect us through inhalation or being massage into the skin.

The same essential oil can have one effect when it is being inhaled and a different affect when it is massaged into the skin.

Peppermint or camphor will open up sinus when inhaled. But you can inhale it all you want and it will not have an analgesic effect on sore muscles until it is massaged into the skin.

Most essential oils have very subtle effects. Do not expect that a one time application of essential oils or herbs are going to magically relieve depression, stop tension or even relieve insomnia. They must be used repeatedly throughout the day. They will enhance the ritual of taking a bath or preparing a cup of tea. They will make a massage more effective. Remember they help bring balance. You must also work on the cause. If you are royally pissed off, or just experienced a knock down, drug out fight, there is no herb or essential oil that is going to bring you peace and calm.

You can see more immediate results from the more aggressive essential oils that contain menthol for their cooling effect on pain, or Eucalyptus or Peppermint for sinus decongestion. An extract of Cayenne will have an immediate heating action. Ginger or Peppermint tea may bring quick relief from indigestion or nausea.

It takes 1 acre to make 15-20 pounds of Lavender oil. It takes 60,000 roses to make one ounce of rose oil which makes rose oil the most expensive essential oil you can buy. Essential oils may seem expensive for such tiny bottles, but remember they are concentrated so you only need a few drops at a time.

Use essential oils with caution. Most essential oils cannot be applied directly to the skin but must be diluted with oils, lotions and other carriers. The few exceptions to this are Lavender and Tea Tree. Essential oils may take the finish off of furniture. Keep the bottles away from children. Lavender and Tea Tree may be safe for children in diluted amounts. People can be allergic to certain essential oils just as they are allergic to plants in nature. If you are allergic to cedar trees you are certainly allergic to cedar oil.

Essential oils and fragrant oils are not the same. Fragrances are usually synthetic oil and may cause allergies. Essential oils will state 100 % essential oil on the bottle. If it does not say 100% essential oil it could be a carrier oil with essential oils added to it, or just synthetic fragrances. Fragrant oils or synthetic oils have more varieties to choose from, can many times be more pleasant than essential oils and their fragrance will last much longer than essential oils. Certified Aroma Therapists will argue that a synthetic fragrance cannot be Aroma Therapy. But I point out if that fragrance affects you emotionally is that not aroma therapy? It certainly cannot have a physical effect. But it can have a psychological effect.

All plants do not have essential oils.

Examples of synthetic oils.

Apple, Carnation, Coconut, Lilac, Peach, Rain, Raspberry, Strawberry, Rose that costs less than $50 for 2 ml.

Project supplies needed: bottles of essential oils and fragrance oils labels hidden and coffee beans to clear the scent.

Not considering whether or not it is an essential oil, or a fragrance oil, choose which bottle you enjoy the most.
Is this an essential oil or a fragrance oil?

When choosing essential oils for your clients, keep in mind these oils are being absorbed into your body through your hands. Only offer essential oils that you enjoy and are appropriate for you. Because there are so many oils to choose from there will be no problem finding an oil appropriate for both you and your client.

8 Methods of Using Essential Oils

DISPERSING THROUGH THE AIR

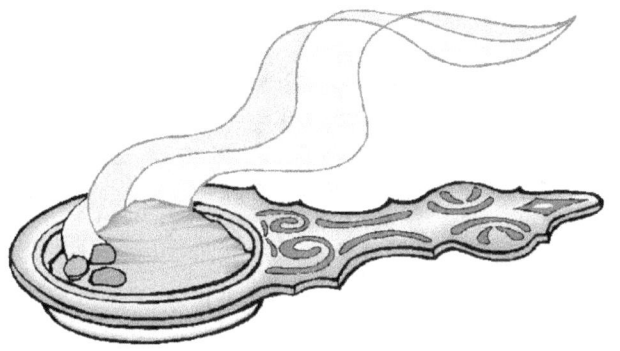

Room Spray

Blend 10 drops of essential oil with 7 tablespoons of water and add 1 tablespoon of Vodka to act as a preservative.

From ancient times in all civilizations, burning of aromatic woods and gums have been used as a fumigant to prevent disease and as an antiseptic. All religions have used some sort of incense for worship and religious ritual.

Essential oils dispersed into the air helps relieve conditions of the respiratory system, the circulatory system and the nervous system.

According to Clinical Aromatherapy by Jane Buckle, research showed that there was a change of brain rhythms within 15 seconds of inhaling certain essential oils, effecting the mood.

Essential oils evaporate quickly. The effect is short lived. Many methods have been devised to keep the oil in the air longer.

Cold Diffusing

Since there is no heat and no chemical propellants the essential oil is not contaminated or altered.

An atomizing diffuser is the most efficient method of diffusing essential oils into the air. The droplets are broken up into a very small mist keeping the oil in the air for several hours. It also has the added benefit of creating a low dose of natural ozone. In large open spaces the diffuser could be kept running all day. In a small room or office, diffuse for 15-30 minutes 3 times a day.

Room spray can be made using water, alcohol, and essential oils. The droplets are sprayed in large droplets and only lasts seconds. If it is sprayed on any kind of fiber the scent would last longer.
Blend 10 drops of essential oil with 7 tablespoons of water, adding 1 tablespoon of Vodka to act a s a preservative.

Blend 40-50 drops of a blend of essential oil to 1 cup of water plus 4 tablespoons of Vodka to act as a preservative.

Shake well before using.

Vaporizers:
The essential oil is dropped on a tissue which is placed over the opening where the steam comes out. It is not poured into the water itself. A combination of Peppermint, Eucalyptus, and Lavender would be good for a cold and congestion.

Hot Diffusion

Hot diffusion vaporizes the essential oil dispersing it through the air. Examples would be a small candle burned under the essential oil, or a small light bulb.

Aromatic Candles:
The least effective way of dispersing essential oils is through candles scented with essential oils. As the wax melts the essential oils are

released through the air and much of the essential oil is consumed by the flame itself. Soot and wax is released into the air. Many candles will have a caution not to burn more than an hour at a time and that the wax and soot may stick to your curtains.

Pretty to look at, pretty to burn, that wax is going somewhere, maybe your lungs.

In choosing which essential oils to disperse into the air, consider the area and the purpose. Is your purpose to cleanse the air, provide some sort of protection against disease, relieve congestion or relax and soothe.
Some suggestions:

Calming: Lavender, Chamomile
Wake up call in the morning: Rosemary, Pine, Mints
Aphrodisiac: Ylang Ylang, Jasmine
Respiratory: Peppermint, Eucalyptus, Lavender, Pine
Antidepressant: Frankincense and Myrrh
Purifer: Lemongrass, Lemon, Pine, Geranium, Oregano
Memory: Basil, Rosemary

Cautions:

Use with caution around people with allergies, emphysema, asthma and newborn babies.
Do not use these essential oil in a diffuser: Thuja, Pennyroyal, Mugwort, Hyssop, Sage, Lavender Stoechas

Through the skin: Massage

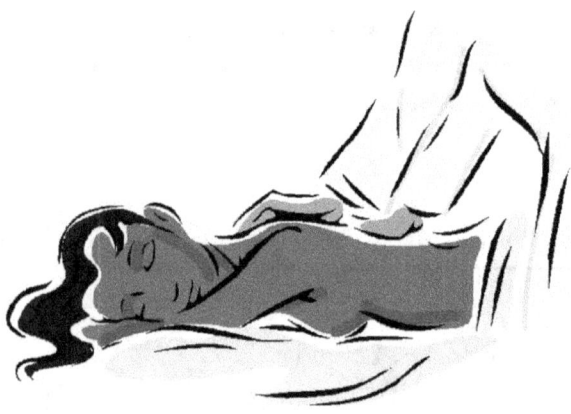

A massage warms up the skin and dilates the blood vessels helping the body absorb the essential oils better and for the oils to penetrate the skin better.

The time it takes for essential oils to be absorbed by the skin and enter the bloodstream will depend on the essential oil, the type of oil carrier, temperature of the body and condition of the skin. All constituents of the essential oil will not enter the bloodstream equally.

If the skin is covered after applying the oils, 75% of the essential is absorbed, if left uncovered only 4% of the essential oil is absorbed. When you turn your client over, you are basically covering up the skin.

Ketones in essential oils will enter the bloodstream within 10 minutes.
Linalol and linalyl acetate 2 main constituents of Lavender are absorbed within 20 minutes and eliminated within 90 minutes.

So how much does that tell you about how long an essential oil would be effective?

How long does a massage effect a person?

Suggested Ratio of Essential Oil to carrier oil for full massage

Physical effect: Up to 30 drops per 1 oz. of carrier oil or 10-15 drops per 4 tablespoons of carrier oil. 1-3 drops per teaspoon of carrier oil. Use less for pregnant women and children, ½ as much.

Scent Only: 10 drops per 1 oz.

If you have spread lotion or oil on your client, you can add essential oils neat since the lotion on your client will dilute the essential oils.

Stronger ratios can be used if massaging one part of the body or for acute conditions confined to one part of the body, such as muscular pain or arthritis.

Project:

Go outside and rub essential oil Peppermint on toes. Cover with socks. Clean hands with alcohol so all traces of the scent of Peppermint will not be in the room. Look at the clock. Determine how many minutes it takes to smell Peppermint or taste the Peppermint.

There is No Problem a Bath Can't Fix!

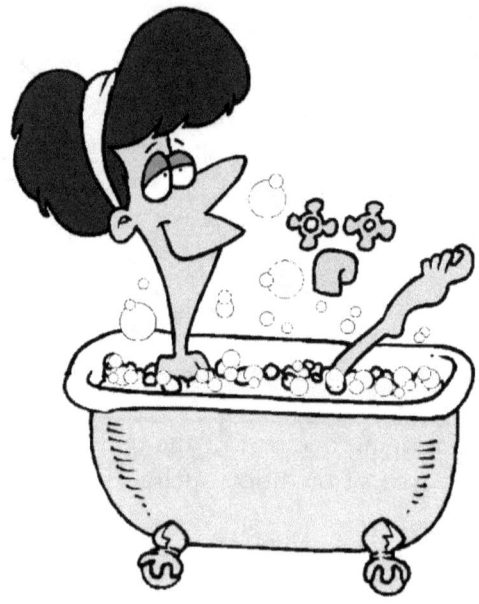

A shower may get you really clean, but a bath can be so many things,
Escape for just a little while, from life's demands and shattered dreams,
A bath can often bring relief from broken hearts and body parts,
A bath can wash away the hurt, a shower can only clean the dirt.

Carolyn Gibson

Taking a bath is one of the most effective ways of absorbing essential oils.

Essential Oils do not mix with water. They will float on top of the water and can irritate sensitive areas on contact. Always mix essential oils with a carrier such as ¼ cup of salt, bath salts or crystals, ½ oz. of milk, egg yolks, honey, unscented liquid soap, unscented bath gels, and carrier oils. Use caution when mixing with carrier oils as this will make your tub slippery. Generally use 5-20 drops of essential oils per bath. Use the lesser amount with aggressive oils such as Peppermint. More than 5 drops of Peppermint may cause hypothermia. Other aggressive oils may have other ill effects. Once when I had a cold I added 30 drops of my sinus congestion mixture of Peppermint, Eucalyptus, and Lavender to my bath. I became extremely cold and had to go to bed with a heating pad to get warmed up.

Cautions for Essential Oils

Essential oils are not normally taken orally or applied directly to the skin

except for a few exceptions.

Other Cautions Below

Oral ingestion

Essential oils are not normally taken internally unless you have had medical training in essential oils. There are a few exceptions that are generally safe. Oils that you would normally use in cooking can be taken internally if they are diluted.

Nausea or digestion: a few drops of essential oil of Peppermint added to a sugar cube or honey. Peppermint candy is basically sugar with essential oil of Peppermint.

Stuffy nose:
When the nose is so stuffed up and breathing essential oils can't get through try 3 drops of essential oil of Peppermint added to 2 tablespoons of honey. Mix well. Place a small amount on the tongue. The molecules of the essential oil of Peppermint can go behind the pharynx into the nasal cavities as a decongestant.
Longer action: add Peppermint to honeycomb as a natural chewing gum.

Antispasmodic:
Add 1 drop of essential oil of Basil to 1 spoonful of honey added to hot water and drank as a tea.

Sore throat:
4 drops of Tea Tree Oil added to 1 tablespoon of honey. Use a pea size on the tongue. Or
One drop on the finger, remove excess on opening of bottle, place on tongue. Apply ever minute for ten minutes.

Neat Application

The term neat means that you can apply the essential oil directly to the skin. Do not use essential oils without diluting them except for these exceptions, Lavender and Tea Tree. These others can be used neat on persons who are not sensitive. Do the foot test if you have sensitive skin, for children under 2, and for pregnant women. Apply to bottom of feet. If skin feels irritated apply vegetable oil to dilute the essential oil.

True Lavender, Tea Tree, Helichrysum, Geranium Graveolens, Carrot Seed, Cedarwood, Celery Seed, Chamomile both Roman and German, Fennel, Galbanum, Jasmine, Myrrh, Neroli, Patchouli, Petigrain, Rose, Rosewood, Sandalwood, Spiknard, Blue Tansy, Valerian Root, Vetiver, Yarrow, Ylang,Ylang, and Peppermint if the individual does not have sensitive skin.

True Lavender (Lavandula angustifolia) is generally safe for all conditions. Burns, cuts, insect bites, scrapes and down the neck for headache stress.

Tea Tree
Apply neat for fungal infections, sores in mouth, and insect bites.

Peppermint Oil:
Headaches; apply to temple, forehead and behind the ears. ***Do not use on children for headache.***
Hiccups: Apply on each side of 5th cervical vertebrae.

Pain caused by a hit or a blow, use immediately to create a cold effect on non sensitive areas of the body. If the body is cut or there is a sore use around the area but not on it.

Helichrysum with Lavender
Use to prevent bruising after pain has been relieved with Peppermint.

Geranium gravelolens:
Stop bleeding on small cuts by applying a few drops to a cotton ball, place cotton ball on cut and apply pressure for 1 minute. Cover with plastic wrap for 12 hours.

Other Cautions and Advice

Always have a good quality vegetable oil for dilution. Water will not dilute an essential oil.

If the oil is accidentally rubbed in the eye blot the eyes with a cotton ball with almond oil if you have it or a good quality vegetable oil.

Do not use essential oils on sensitive area or mucous membranes. Dilute with vegetable oil.

If swallowed take 1-2 tablespoons of virgin vegetable oil.
In case of particular dangerous essential oils such as Sage, Thuja, Pennyroyal, and Hyssop use activated charcoal.

Do not use essential oils such as Peppermint that are high in menthol around the necks of children under 30 months.

Aggressive Essential Oils

Dilute these oils 1 part essential oil to 4 parts carrier oil:
Cassia, Cinnamon Bark, Clove, Hyssop, Lemongrass, Oregano, Peppermint (except for pain in non sensitive areas) Thyme,

Essential Oils that are photosensitive (do not use if you will be in direct sunlight or using tanning beds, or other ultra violet lights.)
Angelica, Bergamot, German Chamomile, all the citrus essential oils:
Citrus Hystrix, Grapefruit, Lemon, Lime, Orange, Tangerine,

Cautions:
Thuja, Pennyroyal, Mugwort, Hyssop, Sage, Lavender Stoechas

Do not use essential oil on clients undergoing chemotherapy without physicians permission.

Do not use while pregnant:
Basil, Calamus Root, Camphor, Carrot Seed, Cedarleaf, Cedarwood, Cinnamon, Ginger, Juniper Berry, Myrrh, Nutmeg, Rosemary, Sage, Vetiver, Wormwood

9 Learning From the Pros

You are not going to become an Aromatherapist in a one day class. You can make intelligent choices. You can look at the ingredients of commercially made products and see what they are combining together. Some therapeutic products will list the essential oils and then list the benefit of each.

Read these labels from Biofreeze, main ingredient is menthol.

Sombra or Sore No More:
Essential oils used would be menthol from Peppermint, Camphor from the Camphor tree. Rest of the ingredients are extracts. Capsaicin which comes from peppers, Queen of the Prairie extract, a source of salicylic acid which was the original ingredient in aspirins before aspirins were made from synthetic ingredients.

Genacol
The essential oil in this is Wintergreen.

Spa products can be deceiving. If you look at these bottles of Biotone customizing complex you will read essential oils, and extracts of and some say Aromatic Blend.
What is the Aromatic Blend? Is this a fragrance?

I do not know. I cannot find an answer to this question. But my customers do love the scent of these.

Other bottles of their customizing complexes do not state Aromatic Blend.

Relaxing Blend:
Lavender, Calendula, Rosewood, Orange, Hops, Cinnamon, Blue Malva, Evening Primrose. Evening Primrose would be a carrier oil and not an essential oil.

Sore Muscle:
Rosemary, Juniper, Lavender, Peppermint, Eucalyptus, Rosewood, Orange, Ginger, Black Pepper

Uplifting:
Verbena, Grapefruit, Lemongrass, Orange, Bergamot, Rosewood

Detoxifying:
Rosemary, Burdock, Echinacea, Lemon, Figwort, Watercress, Geranium, Coriander, Orange, Eucalyptus

Project:
Look on the internet. Can you find essential oil of Burdock or Echinacea?

How about essential oil of Figwort?

Does using this many oils in each formula make them more effective? Or is this copyright or trademark protection?

In this book Aromatherapy by Roberta Wilson, she uses 5-6 oils in each formula. I don't know if that is to making the formula more effective or just making the formula copyright protected.

The book The Essential Aromatherapy Book recommends only blending 3 oils at a time to keep from distracting from each oils individual quality. If your desire is to create your own formulas and not use the commercially prepared products, this will be much more cost effective.

I do not like to use the pain ointments in my massage because it interferes with the glide of the massage lotions. It is just much easier to add my own essential oils or herbal oils to the lotion I am using.

I do like to use the commercially prepared oils if I am just wanting to give my clients a scented massage that they will enjoy.

If I want to compliment the massage with a custom blend, that I can also make body products to send home with the customer, then I am going to use the affordable essential oils with inexpensive supplies.

MY FAVORITE COMBINATIONS ARE:

Geranium and Patchouli
Geranium reduces cortisone hormones in the blood, increases endorphins, relieves anxiety and increases vitality.
Patchouli is said to be a sedative for the soul.

Lavender and Ylang Yylang
Lavender is considered the universal oil that is safe enough for everyone, has a calming effect on the central nervous system, and is a sedative.
Ylang Ylang has a calming effect, relaxes, and is also a sedative.

An essential I like to use by itself is **Frankincense.**
Frankincense causes deep breathing, important for a massage, and will help me slow down while doing a massage especially if I have been rushing around prior to the massage.
Frankincense is also an anti-inflammatory and good for respiration and depression.

Peppermint, Lavender and Eucalyptus
I end a massage session with this combination. The Peppermint and Eucalyptus should enter through the feet to help unstop their noses and stimulate them to wake up. The Lavender softens the blend.

Ylang Ylang, Marjoram, Rosemary
This gentle aroma is for those experiencing sorrow. Ylang Ylang is a potent relaxant that is also stimulating. Egyptians used Marjoram to comfort mourners. The Europeans used Rosemary to help overcome grief. 2 parts Marjoram, 1 part Rosemary, 6 parts Ylang Ylang

10 Essential Oils and Common Remedies

These remedies are for treating small areas using therapeutic grade essential oils. These recommendations are for adults. Dilute twice as much for those that are sensitive. Do not use on pregnant women or children. The dilution is stronger than normally recommended. Use with discretion.

Muscles and Joints: *Combine 1 part of essential oils with 1 part carrier oil, apply 4-6 drops of the combination on effected area 2-3 times daily. Blend up to 3 essential oils except where noted.*

Aches and Pain:
Chamomile Roman or German, Coriander, Eucalyptus, Helichrysum, Ginger, Lavender, Peppermint, Black Pepper, Rosemary, Sage, Wintergreen

Arthritis:
Chamomile Roman or German, Eucalyptus, Ginger, Black Pepper, Lavender, Pine, Rosemary, Spruce

Headache:1 part essential oil to 1 part carrier oil, apply 1-3 drops of combination on back of neck, behind ears, temples, forehead and under nose. Inhalation: 15 minutes 3-5 times a day.
Basil, Chamomile Roman or German, Eucalyptus, Fennel, Geranium, Lavender, Lemon Balm (Melisa), Mint; Peppermint or Spearmint, Rosemary, Wintergreen

Mix a few drops of essential oil of Peppermint with a pea size of honey and place on tongue.

Inflammation, Cartilage Injury, Ligament Sprain or Tear, Tendonitis, Combine 1 part of essential oils with 1 part carrier oil, elevate and apply ice packs, 15 minutes at a time.
Benzoin, Black Pepper, Cedar, Chamomile, Clary Sage, Coriander, Dill, Fennel, Frankincense, Ginger, Helichrysum, Lavender, Peppermint, Pettigrain, Marjoram, Sage, Valerian, Wintergreen

Inflammation due to bruising and tissue damage; Myrrh and Lavender, equal parts essential oil to carrier oil apply twice a day

Inflammation caused by bacterial infection: German Chamomile and Tea Tree: equal parts essential oil to carrier oil apply twice a day

Inflammation caused viral infection: Ravensara, Hyssop, and Thyme 1 part essential oil to 4 parts carrier oil applied 2 times a day

Muscular Cramps and Stiffness: Equal parts EO to Carrier Oil
Allspice, Basil, Black Pepper, Lavender, Peppermint, Sweet Marjoram, Rosemary, Tarragon

Menstrual Cramps: Equal parts EO to Carrier Oil

Basil, Chamomile, Cypress, Helichrysum, Marjoram, Ylang Ylang

Muscle Tension: Equal parts EO to Carrier Oil
Chamomile, Helichrysum, Lavender, Marjoram

Sprains and Strains: Equal parts EO to Carrier Oil
Chamomile Roman and German, Lavender, Sweet Marjoram

Sore Muscles: Biotone : Equal parts EO to Carrier Oil
Rosemary, Juniper, Lavender, Peppermint, Eucalyptus, Rosewood, Sweet Orange, Ginger, Black Pepper

Circulation

Edema and Water Retention: Equal parts EO to Carrier Oil Massage from feet to ankles up, to the thigh, light strokes. 3-5 drops 2-3 times a day.
Angelica, White Birch, Carrot Seed, Cypress, Sweet Fennel, Geranium, Grapefruit, Juniper Berry, Lovage, Patchouli, Tangerine, Wintergreen

Suggested Blend to add to equal parts carrier oil
10 drops Wintergreen, 8 drops Tangerine, 6 drops Sweet Fennel, 4 drops Juniper Berry, 3 drops Patchouli

Caution: Keep in mind contraindications: heart conditions and high blood pressure. The heart pumps the fluid, is the heart strong enough to handle the extra work.
Consider the cause: Diuretics to flush the kidneys, possible potassium deficiency, drink more water, elevate the effected body part.

Gout:
Angelica, Carrot seed, Juniper, Lemon, Roman Chamomile, Rosemary, Tea Tree

Gout blend to apply neat: 10 drops of Lemon, 4 drops Juniper Berry, 3 drops of tea tree , 2 drops of Roman Chamomile.

Digestion
Enteric-coated capsules of the essential oil of peppermint is effective for irritable bowel syndrome.

Nausea or Motion sickness: Equal parts of essential oil to carrier oil, 1-3 drops of combination applied behind each ear, and over navel 2-3 times hourly. Inhalation: Patchouli, Peppermint

Apply Peppermint to tongue 1-4 times as needed.

Ear Aches: Never put essential oils into the ear canal. Apply around the opening.
Mix equal amounts of these essential oils with warm olive oil or coconut oil: Place 2 drops on a cotton swab and apply to the skin around the ear opening or 2 drops on a cotton ball and place over the ear opening. Optional: Warm Compress over the ear.
Niaouli, Wintergreen, Tea Tree, Lavender, Rosemary, Roman Chamomile, Helichrysum, Peppermint, Eucalyptus

Ears, Tinnitus
1-2 drops of Helichrysum applied neat on temples, forehead, back of neck, 1 drop on tip of toes and fingers.

Mix equal amounts of essential oils and carrier oils and apply to temples, forehead, and back of neck.
Basil, Geranium, Juniper berries, Lavender, Peppermint

Eye Problems: never put essential oils near or into the eyes.
Dilute 1 part essential oil to 4 parts of carrier oil.
Apply 2-4 drops of diluted essential oil blend 1-3 times a day. Make a wide circle around the eyes, above the eyebrows, across the temples and under the cheeks ending at the bridge of the nose. If you accidentally get essential oils into eyes, flush with vegetable oil, never water.

Clove, Lavender, Lemon, Cypress, Eucalyptus radiate

Eye Blend for cataracts: 10 drops lemon, 5 drops Cypress, 3 drops Eucalyptus radiate. Add 1 part of essential oil blend to 4 parts carrier oil. **Remember wide circle around the eyes, not in the eyes.**

Pink eye: **Remember wide circle around the eyes, not in the eyes.**
Tea Tree, Lavender

Fibromyalgia: Mix equal parts of essential oils to 1 part carrier oil, apply 2-4 drops and massage into effected area. Warm compresses on effected area
Frankincense, Wintergreen,
Blend: 8 drops of Balsam Fir, 6 drops of White Fir, 4 drops Wintergreen, 2 drops Spruce

Lice: Equal Parts of Essential Oil to Carrier Oil, massage 1 teaspoon of oil blend into scalp. Cover with plastic shower can and leave on for at least 30 minutes. Shampoo and rinse well.
Tea Tree, Thyme, Lavender, Geranium

Lice Blend: 2 drops of Geranium, 2 drops of lemon, and 4 drops of Thyme.

The Nervous System

Use in Baths, As Inhalation and Massage

Anxiety
Basil, Lemon Balm, Bergamot, Chamomile, Cypress, Geranium, Jasmine (not an essential oil but an absolute) Frankincense, Lavender, Neroli, Patchouli, Rose, Rosewood, Clary Sage, Sage, Sandalwood, Ylang, Ylang

Depression:
Basil, Bergamot, Chamomile, Cypress, Geranium, Jasmine (not an essential oil an absolute), Lavender, Orange Blossom (Neroli), Patchouli, Rose, Sandalwood, Ylang Ylang

Insomnia
Lemon Balm, Chamomile Roman or German, Hops, Lavender, Linden, Orange Blossom(Neroli), Valerian,

Mental Fatigue:
Basil, Juniper, Lemon Balm (Melissa), Pine, Rosemary Sage, Clary Sage, Thyme

Migraine:
Lavender, Mint Peppermint or Spearmint

Nervous Exhaustion:
Angelica, French Basil, Mint Peppermint or spearmint, Rosemary, Clary Sage, Spanish Sage, Vetiver

Nervous Tension and Stress:
Lemon Balm, Bergamot, Chamomile Roman or German, Frankincense, Hops, Lavender, Linden, Sweet Marjoram, Orange Blossom (Neroli), Patchouli, Rose, Clary Sage, Sandalwood, Veviter, YlangYlang

Neuralgia, Sciatica:
Chamomile Roman or German, Spike Lavender, Sweet Marjoram, Rosemary

Relaxing: Biotone
Lavender, Calendula, Rosewood, Orange, Hops, Cinnamon, Blue Malva,

Shock:
Lemon Balm, Orange Blossom

Uplifting: Biotone
Verbena, Grapefruit, Lemongrass, Orange, Bergamot, Rosewood

As you can see there are many essential oils to choose from. Take notice of the essential oils that have multiple healing properties. For economic reasons, choose a few that serve multiple purposes and that speak to you. Learning as much as you can about a few essential oils rather than boggling your mind with many will make your choice of essential oils more effective.

11 Complimentary Products

Aromatherapy can create an emotional connection between you and your clients by bringing you to mind when they take home complimentary products using the same scent that was used in your massage session or scents that are in the air of your reception area.

From hand creams to lip balm they begin with your homemade herbal oil.
Choose glass or stainless steel, or enameled containers, never use aluminum or non- stick coated pans.
I find that the permanent basket style re-usable coffee filters make the best strainers.

First choose your oil using cold pressed oils. Odena used canola oil straight from the grocery store. After becoming a massage therapist and learning the value of the right oil I chose Safflower oil.

Safflower oil contains essential fatty acids to help damaged skin.
Grapeseed oil is light and non-greasy good for massage.
Apricot, avocado, and sunflower oils are also good.
Olive oil is used because it will not go rancid as quick.
Jojoba is the most expensive of the oils does not require refrigeration and will not go rancid.
Old herbals used mineral oil and petroleum jelly. Even baby oil was made with mineral oil. It was cheap, readily available and no one was likely to have allergies to it. Remember that mineral oil is a petroleum product. Do you really want that on your skin?

Coconut oil **is not good** to use by itself because it will get rock hard if the temperature is below 70 degrees.

Comfrey or Lemon Balm Oil: Using fresh herbs

1 quart of fresh Comfrey leaves and roots if available or 1 quart of fresh Lemon Balm leaves
1 quart of cold pressed oil of your choice. I use safflower oil.

Combine chopped leaves and the oil in a large baking dish, bake in oven at under 200°f 2-3 hours or until leaves are crispy. If after 3 hours the leaves are still not crispy turn your temperature up 25 degrees. Let cool slightly and strain. You do not want to melt your strainer.
An alternative method would be to heat gently on top of the stove, keeping the temperature below 200 °F. Again, Odena cooked hers on top of the stove. To me it is easier to keep the temperature under 200°f in the oven than watching it on top of the stove.

The oil will be easier to strain and pour if it is still warm as it tends to thicken up when cool and will not go through the strainer as well. Pour the strained oil into a container, I use the bottle that the cold pressed oil came in.

For each 4 oz of oil add 1 vitamin E capsule or ¼ teaspoon if your vitamin E is in a bottle.
If you are using your oil to use as an herbal oil only, you can add your essential oil to the whole bottle.

Or bottle up in smaller bottles and customize the blend by adding essential oils individually.
For each 1 oz. of oil add 10-30 drops of essential oil.

If you are using your oil to make lotions, salves or balms wait and add your essential oils to the final product.

I store my herbal oil in the refrigerator and pour a small amount into a small eye dropper bottle that I can leave out on the counter for daily use.

Herbal Oil Using dried herbs.

Grind 2 ounces of dried herbs and combine with 1 pint (2 cups) of your chosen cold pressed oil.

Heat the oil and herbs either on top of the stove or in the oven under 200°F for one hour. Strain and pour into bottle.
For each 4 oz of oil add 1 vitamin E capsule or ¼ teaspoon if your vitamin E is in a bottle.

Salves and Balms

Salves and balms are basically oil with beeswax added as a thickener and for its healing properties. Salves and Balms are thick and are made to stay on the skin longer. 1 oz. of beeswax is added to 1 cup of herbal oil or a salve or lip gloss and 2 ounces of beeswax for lip balms that go into tubes.

If you buy a block of beeswax you will find it nearly impossible to cut or scrape to measure the 1 tablespoon or ounces that you need. Buy the beeswax beads to save time and frustration. If your recipe calls for 1 oz. of beeswax then buy the beeswax in 1 oz. bars.

Lotions and Creams have water or other liquids added to the mix and are thinner. They evaporate fairly quick.

First Aid Salve or Lip Balm

Comfrey or Lemon Balm Lip Balm or Salve
1-2 tablespoon of beeswax (see note below)
2 teaspoons of honey
5 tablespoons of herbal oil
20 drops of essential oil

Heat 5 tablespoons of your herbal oil with 1 tablespoon of beeswax slowly until it reaches 160°f. Remove from heat and add honey and blend together. Fill either lip balm tubes or small containers1/2 full.

Put 1 drop of essential oil into container. Fill again and then add 1 more drop of essential oil. Then top off if the tube is not full. Using 1 tablespoon of beeswax makes a softer balm more suitable for the 3 ml containers. 2 tablespoons of beeswax is better for the tubes. Makes about 20 tubes or 20 3 ml containers.

Beeswax Moisturizing Cream

is adapted from the recipe by Linda Pelham of the East Texas Beekeepers Association. She uses mineral oil or baby oil, I use the Comfrey Oil or Lemon Balm Oil.

Your clients will love this to moisturize, calm skin irritations, insect bites, stings, and itching. It is good from head to toe. It feels a little sticky when you first put it on but dries quickly and becomes silky smooth.

Comfrey Beeswax Moisturizing Cream
6 oz of Comfrey oil
2 oz. of beeswax (weigh with scales)
8 oz of distilled water
2 teaspoons of Borax
2 containers for heating, postage scale or other scale for weighing beeswax, 2 instant read thermometers, timer, 2 whisks
Recipe makes about 16 ounces.

Heat on low to medium heat the herbal oil and beeswax slowly until it reaches 160°F. Container needs to be big enough to hold at least 4 cups. This may take 30-40 minutes.

Pour Borax into a heat proof measuring cup (at least 2 cups) Heat the water in a separate pan until it reaches 160°F and pour into the cup with the Borax and whisk until dissolved.

Pour the water and Borax into the pan with the oil and beeswax. Stir continuously with a whisk for 5 minutes or until the mixture reaches a temperature of 140°f. Use the timer. The last 30 seconds stir slowly to eliminate bubbles. Pour the cream into containers. Let it cool a little more and add your essential oils. For each 1 oz. of cream add 30 drops of essential oil. Stir the essential oil inside the container before it starts to thicken. Do not put lid on until cream has completely cooled.

***All natural Hand and Body Lotion from Starwest Wholesale
A little thinner than the Beeswax Moisturizing Cream***

1 cup of Starwest Aloe Vera Gel
1 teaspoon of Starwest lanolin
1 teaspoon of vitamin E oil
1/3 cup of Starwest coconut oil
¼ ounce of Starwest beeswax (this is .25 on a digitial scale)
¾ cup of Starwest sweet almond oil or grapeseed oil
1-2 teaspoons of Starwest essential or fragrance oils of your choice.
I used 1 teaspoon of Lavender and thought this was much too
strong) optional: 1 dropperful of bee propolis

Combine the beeswax, and coconut oil in a 2 cup heat proof
measuring cup. Microwave on high for 30 seconds and stir. Repeat
in ten second intervals until the beeswax and oil is fully melted
(I would never microwave an item I thought was being used for
healing properties). I would heat on low heat to 160ºF.

Mix the Almond or Grapeseed oil into the mixture. (I used my
comfrey oil) Reheat if necessary.
 Pour the Aloe Vera gel, the lanolin, and the vitamin E into blender
or food processor and blend on low or medium.

Stream the melted oils into the blender. As the oils blend together
the mixture will turn white and the motor will start to grind. Stop
when the motor start to grind and the mixture has the consistency of
mayonnaise .

Add essential oils or fragrance oils and pulse blend.
Pour into containers and screw on lids.

I found this formula to be a bit greasy, it may have been because I
used the comfrey oil instead of the Grapeseed oil or the almond oil.
It did leave my skin feeling silky smooth once it dried.

It also was thinner than the mayonnaise consistency, but once again that may have been because I used my comfrey oil instead of the Grapeseed oil or the almond oil.

Frankincense and Myrrh Honey Pat

2 teaspoon of honey
1 drop of Frankincense essential oil
1 drop of Myrrh essential oil
(any of your favorite essential oils for the skin can be used.)

Pat the honey on the face. The honey will bead up on your face like water beads up on a car. Relax for 10 minutes.
Optional: Place tea bags on your eyes as you relax.

Pat your face with your fingertips for 5 minutes.
Rinse with warm water. Follow with a splash of cold water and then moisturize.

Honey is considered a humectant, meaning it pulls moisture from the air. A honey mask softens and moisturizes dehydrated or flaky skin. It is a light facial peeler removing the outer layer of dead skin and surface blemishes. Honey is naturally acidic so a toner is not needed.

Frankincense and Myrrh are known to rejuvenate mature skin by encouraging new cells to develop.

Sugar or Salt Scrubs:

2 parts of sugar (white or brown)
1 part cold pressed oil or herbal oil
½ teaspoon of vitamin E
Essential oils of choice.

Do not use scrubs on sensitive skin or skin with broken capillaries. Do not use sugar and salt scrubs on the face.. Use stimulating essential oils on the feet, hands, and limbs. Use relaxing essential oils on the chest and neck.

CONTINUE YOUR THEME WITH YOUR CUSTOMIZE SCENTED FOAMING HAND SOAP

Foaming hand soap is all about the container and pump not the soap. A foaming pump will make any liquid soap foaming hand soap.

The secret is the ratio of liquid soap to water. Dr. Bronner liquid castile soap is natural and safe for all persons.
Use a ratio of 60% of liquid soap to 40% distilled water or bottled water. Concentrated liquid soaps you buy from suppliers for the soap foamers will give you their ratio.
Then add your customize blend of essential oils.

Make scented candles and scented soap with your customized blend of essential oils.

Candles are simple to make with the right supplies and instructions.

Making soap can be quite time consuming and require room to let them set and age.

Thankfully there are melt and pour soaps that you can add your customized blend of essential oils.

Dressing up your Complimentary Products, Bottles and Tins

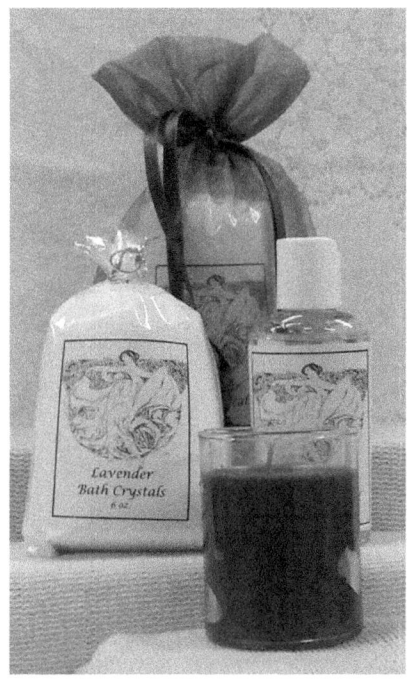

Imagine a floral fragrance draining your body of anger, resentments and old hurts.

Imagine,

Letting Go.

When working with essential oils or fragrant oils you must use containers that have a vapor lock. Otherwise your scent will evaporate through the container in as little as a week's time. You cannot use zip lock bags or other such plastic bags you buy at the grocery store.

Either use glass containers, tin containers or cello bags.
Cello bags are available in small amounts at places such as Hobby Lobby and Michael's, normally found in the candy and cake section.

For larger quantities order from the supplier list you will find below.

Ribbons, boxes, metal ties, etc will make your products look professional.

Use copyright free clip art to dress up your products. I use Dover Publications and Art Explosion. Office supply has many shapes and sizes of labels that you can choose for your products and insert clip art into. If you cannot find the right size label buy the full page label and cut to fit.

Pipettes are invaluable in working with essential oils and fragrance oils. They are used for measuring your oils and dispensing your oils. It is almost impossible to measure oils accurately by shaking them from a standard bottle of essential oil.

If you are poetic use your talent to name and describe your products or your treatments.

You have my permission to use these copyright verses on your product labels, or describing a treatment, but may not reproduce in a book, or other publications without giving me credit. Feel free to change the essential oil blends.

Sample of my labels:
Letting Go
Imagine a floral fragrance draining your body of anger, resentments and old hurts. Imagine Letting Go.
Essential oil of Lavender and Ylang Ylang. Lavender is one of the most well known herbs used to treat anxiety. It has a long history of effecting deep relaxation. Brain wave test proved Lavender to have the greatest sedative effect of all the herbs tested.

A Time for Sorrow:
Allow the gentle aroma to surround you, comfort you, and fill your empty heart. .
Use these oils to comfort you through your time of loss, rather it be the loss of a loved one, a job, or a relationship or maybe when you have just lost your joy.
This blend contains the costly essential oils of YLang Ylang, Marjoram, and Rosemary. Ylang Ylang is a potent relaxant that is also stimulating. Egyptians and Greeks used Marjoram to comfort mourners. The Europeans used Rosemary to help overcome grief.

Up-Lifting
When there are more disappointments than you can handle, or it just seems things are never going to get any better, allow the penetrating aroma to UP-Lift your soul, giving you a hope for a better tomorrow.
Essential oils of Ylang Ylang, Lavender, Sweet Orange

Sometimes synthetic fragrances , although not natural and not healing can be used just for the enjoyment of the scent in a bath or as a perfume. One of my favorites from Mike's Fragrances n More is Sex on the Beach. I changed the name to On the Beach, just because I didn't want the word sex associated with my practice.

On the Beach
Remember times, or were those dreams? Of loving, laughing on the beach.

Another one is Egyptian Musk. I changed the name to Subtle Pleasures.

Subtle Pleasures
Pamper yourself in a subtle fragrance suggesting love and other pleasures. Experience the sensual aroma, forgetting to resist…

12 Resources and the Texas Resale Certificate

Obtaining a Texas Resale Certificate will open up doors to you in adding to your profit margin. As a Texas Massage Therapist you are a business. Maybe you do not have your own shop. The state of Texas does not care. Most wholesalers just require a sales tax number. Some wholesalers may require you to have a storefront, when selling items that have a protected market. A resale certificate will get you into some wholesale conventions.

If you are shopping and see an item you think you might like to sell, just contact the manufacture or distributor on the tag, and see what their wholesale requirements are and the minimums. You may need to fill out a business form. Most of them will take credit cards.

Having a Texas Resale Certificate does come with responsibilities. Failing to file each tax period has a fine. Penalties can be high for not claiming income. If you go to different locations outside your city of business you will have to claim and file for each city that you go into, such as fairs and festivals. Many have a different tax rate.

All taxable items have to pay the state sales tax. Depending on the location where you are conducting business , there may or may not be a city sales tax, a county sales tax or other sales tax for special taxing authorities.

You will be provided with a book that supplies tax rates for ever zip code that you do business in.

http://www.window.state.tx.us

These are a few resources, you can check the internet for many others.

If you live in East Texas Mike' Fragrance N More is a local resource for fragrances, some essential oils, bottles, lotion containers, glassware, candle making supplies, soap making supplies, beeswax in bead form, incense and holders.
Mike's Fragrance N More
http://www.mikesfragrancesnmore.com

1601 W Front St.
Tyler TX   75702
903 944 7912

Starwest Botanicals, Inc
http://www.Starwest-Botanicals.com
1 800 800 4372

This is a wholesale supplier that you will need a Texas Resale Certificate. They have a low minimum of $50.00 for a first time order. No minimum after that. They have quality essential oils, some organic, herbs, extracts, teas, etc.

Wholesale Supplies Plus.com
http://www.wholesalesuppliesplus.com
1 800 359 0944
This has the pump and bottle foamers and the tubes for lip balm.

Essential Supplies
http://www.essentialsupplies.com
562 802-0515

Nashville Wraps
http://www.nashvillewraps.com
800 547 9727

13 Supplements for Pain and Inflammation

Inflammation is the body's natural response when we are injured. The symptoms are redness, swelling, heat and pain. Inflammation will cause the blood vessels to dilate bringing in fresh blood with other chemicals to control pathogens and to remove damaged debris. This is natural and part of the healing process.

When we are not injured, and the inflammation is brought on by stress, eating the wrong foods, exercise, or auto immune disease such as arthritis we try and control the inflammation because it is painful. We can take pills, chemical or herbs that will block the chemical messengers in the body signaling the inflammatory response.

Which of these over the counter medications is not an anti-inflammatory?

Ibroprofen, Aspirin, Tylenol

Ice works against inflammation because it constricts the blood vessels restricting blood flow into the area.

http://www.osteobiflex.com

Look at this bottle of Osteo Bio-flex. Can anyone guess what is the secret ingredient in the 5-Loxin of their Joint Shield?

5-LOXIN® Advanced is a super concentrated extract of Boswellia serrata, which helps with joint flare-ups.* Boswellia serrate is Frankincense.

Which ingredient is treating the cause?

_____

Which ingredient is treating the symptom?

_____

http://www.perluxan.com

Perluxan come from which herb?

_____

Which over the counter pain reliever is it compared to?

Which side effect of hops does this not have?

_____

How does Perluxan block pain?

_____

Does Perluxan work faster or slower than Osteo Bioflex?

_____

Click on the link below. Print turmeric in the search bar.

http://www.drweil.com

Turmeric is in what common food?

_____

Turmeric blocks what enzyme to reduce inflammation?

_____

Go back to the above link and click on anti inflammatory diet.

Name 3 foods on the anti inflammatory food pyramid.

_____

A consideration in deciding between natural anti inflammatory is to take in consideration if they are a stimulant or relaxing.

Turmeric is a stimulant, any herb that increases circulation would be a stimulant. What about Frankincense?

If you were going to take an inflammatory at bed time which would you choose?

Go to biofreeze website click on education and then how it works. 5 minute video

http://www.biofreeze.com

_____

What is the active ingredient in Biofreeze?

How does it work?

Cold therapy or heat therapy?

The menthol in Biofreeze creates a sensation that overrides pain signals to the brain. The Gate Control Theory is when one stimulus blocks the pain signals from reaching the brain. Research suggest that menthol also may stimulate the cold receptors in the skin that may also regulate pain.

Sore No More or use to be Sombra

http://sorenomore.com

Name 3 ingredients.

Notice   that none of these products listed essential oil of any herb but listed extracts of.

Which one ingredient do both of these products contain?_____

Name other products that contain menthol._____

What other herb is used as a Gate Control Therapy?

Does cayenne pepper use heat or cold? How does it work differently from cold?

When a pain ointment says it contains menthol, that menthol came from mint. There are several kinds of mints and not all contain menthol.

Other herbs for pain and inflammation. This is in no way a complete list of herbs.

Ashwagandha, Black Cohosh, Cat's Claw, Cayenne, Chamomile, Devil's Claw, Frankincense, Hops, Peppermint, Turmeric, Willow Bark

14 Inflammation and Food

Omega-3 alpha linolenic fatty acid

Research by the top universities show that Omega-3 is essential for healthy brains, lowers the risk of heart disease, arthritis and cancer, fights wrinkles and block fat-cell formation.

We need both Omega 3's and Omega 6's fatty acids in balance for correct blood flow and inflammation. Our American diet consists of too many Omega 6's which creates a deficiency of Omega 3's. Omega 3's promote blood flow and reduces inflammation while Omega 6's promote blood clotting and inflammation.

Omega 3 comes from the green leaves of plants, and from animals that eat green leaves of plants. Ocean fish are a good source of Omega 3 because of they eat phytoplankton and seaweed which are the green leaves of the ocean. Farmed fish are fed corn and soy, therefore are not a good source of Omega 3. Eggs from chickens that eat green leaves are a good source of Omega 3. Farm animals use to be a good source of Omega 3 because they were raised on pasture.

Omega 6 comes from seeds and grains. Now that we are using vegetable oils, such as corn oil and soybean oil we are getting way too many Omega 6's. Chickens are now fed grains, which make their eggs and their meat have more of Omega 6 than Omega 3. Farm animals fed grains have more Omega 6 than Omega 3.

Flaxseed oil, coconut oil and olive oil are good oils with Omega 3.

The author of the Queen of Fats, Susan Allport, believes that the Omega 3's are your spring fats for activity and mating and the

Omega 6's are your storage fats for the winter time for hibernating. The following chart is the conclusion of her research:

Omega 3	Omega 6
Spring Fats	Winter Fats
Source:	Source:
green leaves	seeds and grains
of plants and	and animals
animals that	that eat seeds
eat green leaves	and grains
Speed up	Fat storage for plants
metabolism	Prepares animals for
Prepares us for	hibernation
activity	
Concentrated in	Concentrated in fat of
brains, eyes, heart	plants and animals
tails of sperm	adipose tissue (belly fat of humans

David Perlmutter, MD author of Grain Brain, is passionate in his belief that grains (including whole grain) and high carbohydrate diets (including fruit)   not only causes inflammation but also leads to brain decline and of course diabetes.

15 Essential Oil, Tea, Tincture or Pills?

People are very unique. What works for one does not work for the other. What works for you one time may not work the next time.

Colds, Flu, Sore Throat, Respiratory

First sign of a cold take a tablespoon of *Elderberry Syrup*. Or

Mix *Tea Tree* essential oil with honey. 4 drops of *Tea Tree Oil* added to 1 tablespoon of honey. Use a pea size on the tongue. Or
One drop on the finger, remove excess on opening of bottle, place on tongue. Apply ever minute for ten minutes.

Ginger or Peppermint tea sweetened with honey and lemon.

Bring a cup of chicken soup to a boil, add S*age and Thyme*, turn off the heat and let steep for ten minutes.

Nose Cleansing.
I am sure you have heard of the Neti Pot as a sinus cleansing system. It soothes dry nasal passages, washes away irritants, and helps remove excess mucus. Instead of a Neti Pot I use a syringe (without the needle of course). I found the Neti Pot awkward to use. Using a syringe is so much easier.

Stopped up nose:
Inhale essential oil of *Peppermint* alone or combined with *Eucalyptus* and *Lavender* via a vaporizer or mix with a carrier oil rubbed on the chest or throat.

When the nose is so stuffed up and breathing essential oils can't get through try 3 drops of essential oil of P*eppermint* added to 2 tablespoons of honey. Mix well. Place on the tongue.
The molecules of the essential oil of P*eppermint* can go behind the

pharynx into the nasal cavities as a decongestant.
Longer action: add to honeycomb as a natural chewing gum.

Sore Throat:
Gargle with salt water or *Garden Sage* (Saliva officinalis) tea. Steep 1 teaspoon of dried sage with 1 cup of boiling water. Use as a gargle or add honey and drink as a tea. Add 5 ml of a tincture of Sage to a cup of warm water and drink as a tea or use as a gargle.
Sage Gargle:
Grind 1 oz of dried sage leaves with 1 oz of dried thyme leaves. Cover with 1 quart of apple cider vinegar in a mason jar and stir. Let sit for 2 weeks shaking daily. Strain and put in a dark container. Use as a mouthwash or as a gargle. **Sage is not safe as an essential oil.**

Sore Throat Rub:
Add 5 drops of Rose Scented Geranium to ½ oz of oil

Cough:
Steep 1-2 teaspoon of Thyme in a cup of hot water. Cover the cup so the essentials are not lost. Add honey to taste. Thyme acts as an expectorant and the honey will coat the back of the throat.

Chest Rub:
¼ teaspoon *of Eucalyptus* essential oil
1/8 teaspoon of *Peppermint* essential oil
1/8 Teaspoon *of Thyme* essential oil
¼ cup of olive oil
Add beeswax to make into a salve.

Cold Sores:
Lemon Balm (Melissa officinalis) has research to back up its effectiveness.
A strong tea of Lemon balm can be made and dabbed on the sore 4 times throughout the day. 1-2 Lemon Balm tea bags or 2-4 teaspoons of the dried herb steeped in boiling water 5-10 minutes. Allow to cool before applying with a cotton ball.

Lemon Balm lip balm can be applied 4 times a day. See recipe page 78

If you have cold sores frequently try taking L Lysine. One 500 mg daily to prevent outbreaks and increase to 4 tablets a day if you have an outbreak.

Toothpaste containing sodium lauryl sulfate may cause canker or cold sores.

Insomnia

Herbal tea or herbal tincture:
Chamomile or Lemon balm tea or tincture, mildest, Kava Kava extract or tincture the strongest. Valerian is best taken by pills or capsules as it smells like dirty socks.

Hops can be taken as a tea or a tincture. Hops has estrogen like compounds and should not be taken while pregnant.

An old folk remedy is to make a small pillow of Hops, Lavender and Roses Petals to place in your pillow. Adding Mugwort to this pillow blend is said to make your dreams more vivid.

Essential oil of Lavender is the most well known of the essential oils for insomnia. Rub a few drops on the bottom of your feet, drops can be sprinkled on your pillowcase, or spray the bed with a Lavender Spray, Blend 10 drops of essential oil of Lavender with 7 Tablespoons of water and add 1 tablespoon of Vodka to act as a preservative.

Add essential oils to a hot bath before bedtime. Mix essential oils with a little Epsom Salts, table salt, milk, baking soda or cornstarch. Add a single oil or blend together according to your preference. Lavender by itself, or combined with Ylang Ylang, or combined with Chamomile. Other essential oils for insomnia would be Frankincense, Sandalwood, Rose Scented Geranium.

Mucus:

Another herb I may use instead of Peppermint to help break up mucus is Ginger. I either eat crystallized Ginger or use a high power blender to combine orange juice, oranges, fresh Ginger root and maybe some wheatgrass powder. A good quality Ginger ale will work. In the winter time I will make a Ginger tea, sweetened with honey. If it is really cold outside I may add a little Cayenne pepper.

Muscle Cramps
Pills:
Black Cohosh

Essential Oils:
Basil, Eucalyptus, Peppermint,

Nausea:
Ginger tea, Crystallized Ginger, Ginger Ale, Peppermint tea, Peppermint candy

Pain and Inflammation
Pills , Extracts and rubs
Ashwagandha, Black Cohosh, Cat's Claw, Cayenne, Chamomile, Devil's Claw, Frankincense, Hops, Peppermint, Turmeric, Willow Bark

Essential Oils:
Peppermint Oil for bruises and bumps, Wintergreen, Eucalyptus,

Stop Minor Bleeding:
Apply these to the wound with pressure for a full minute

Rose Scented Geranium drops on a cotton ball applied to injury

Apply fresh Leaves and flowers of *Yarrow* to the wound

Apply Cayenne Pepper powder or tincture to the wound

Vaginal irritations
A sitz bath with Comfrey Root Tea

Wounds and Injuries:
Aloe Vera, Soak in a tea of Comfrey leaves and roots, salves and oil, Echinacea teas, and tinctures

16 My Favorite Herbs

Basil: Ocimim basilicum

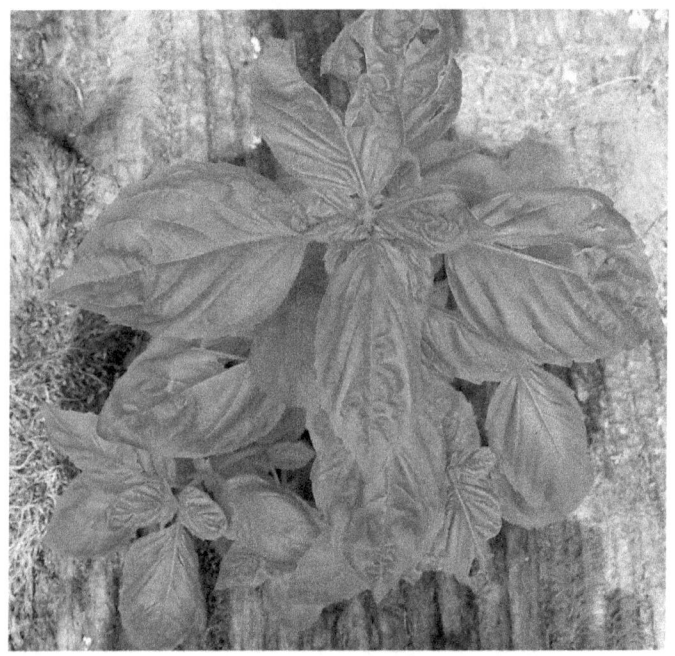

This aromatic herb is a wonderful way to eat healthy. It is high in
vitamins A,C, and anti-oxidants. It is a natural anti-biotic, reduces
nausea from chemotherapy and because it relaxes the intestinal
muscles it helps relieves cramping and gas. Research at the
University of Illinois in Chicago shows that Basil has more than 30
cancer preventing substances. In New Jersey, researchers at Rutgers
University speculate that even a small amount of Basil in your diet
can reduce your risk of cancer.

Basil is used in Malaysia to kill intestinal parasites and used as a stomach soother.

In India, the essential oil of Basil is used to treat acne. A tea or tincture would not be strong enough.

Basil has a reputation for stimulating menstruation, so it should not be used in large quantities by pregnant or nursing women. Culinary amounts are safe.

To make a tea: Pour boiling water (or fruit juice) over 2-3 t of dried leaves or 6 t fresh leaves. Cover and let steep 15-20 minutes. Drink 1 cup for a warm aromatic experience. Drink 3 cups a day for therapeutic benefit.

If using a tincture use 1/2 -1 t 3 times a day.

Pour 1 qt of boiling water over a handful of leaves and steep to use as tea for your bath. Basil is wonderful for the skin or hair.

Basil is best known as a culinary herb. Pesto (an Italian sauce) is Basil's claim to fame. Pasta sauce would not be Italian without Basil.

Add Basil to your salads and vegetables.

There are many varieties of Basil to choose from. The purple Basil makes a beautiful pink vinegar. Once our Texas summer heats up the purple Basil will turn green and if kept cut back will turn purple again once the weather cools off.

Basil is an annual requiring full sunlight and plenty of water. 2 plants should be enough for the average household. If you just love Pesto you might need 6 plants. You need to keep the plant pinched back to promote bushiness and keep it from going to seed. It is sensitive to cold and will stop producing as soon as the weather gets below 50. It will die at first frost. At one time we were the largest organic Basil growers in Texas. Everyone in town knew when I harvested Bail, you could smell me coming.

Cayenne Pepper: Capsicum species

Many times herbs are part of our food chain, such as Cayenne Pepper. The fruit of the plant (the pepper) is the only part of the plant used. Cayenne is one the valuable herbs for circulation. Capsicum, the chemical that makes pepper hot is used in many creams and lotions to treat pain.

Cayenne normalizes circulation, therefore it is safe for persons with either low or high blood pressure. Cayenne can be taken daily as a tonic to help stimulate the heart and circulation. It may even help prevent heart attacks and strokes. Cayenne regulates blood flow, strengthening the heart, arteries, capillaries and nerves.

Because it improves circulation, it is good to take daily for aches and pains. If you have cold hands or feet, that indicates a lack of peripheral circulation. Try Cayenne Pepper.

Cayenne can be used to break up congestion, clear mucus, move blood, help eliminate headaches, cramping and diarrhea. Its stimulating properties increase energy and vitality. Cayenne can help dispel gas, and is good for digestion.

Cayenne Pepper powder can be poured over a wound to stop bleeding (it will not burn the skin).

Take Cayenne at the first sign of a cold, flu, indigestion or if you are just feeling low.

Cayenne is used in herbal formulas to speed the herbs through the body.

There are several ways to take Cayenne internally. The quickest results is Cayenne tea if you can handle really spicy.
Pour 1 cup of boiling water over ¼ - 1 teaspoon of Cayenne powder. Let steep 10 minutes. Add 1 tablespoon of this tea to 1 cup of hot water and drink throughout the day.

Capsules:
An average dose is 2 capsules 3 times a day. You can work up to 3 capsules 3 times a day.
If you have a weak stomach it would be better to start with 1 capsule 3 times a day and see how it works for you.

Try Cayenne Pepper tinctures.

Too much at one time can make you nauseous.

Cayenne Pepper powder or tincture will help stop bleeding.

Of course you can just eat the pepper.

Cayenne Pepper grows well here in East Texas. Cayenne requires regular watering and will even do well in partial shade. All peppers are ripe when they turn red. Even jalapeno and bell peppers are unripe when they are eaten green.

Although Cayenne pepper can be dried on the vine for kitchen use, dry in the shade for therapeutic use.

Ripe Cayenne Pepper is a source of Vitamins A, B1, B2, B3, B5, B6, B9 and vitamin C.

Avoid Cayenne if you are prone to nosebleeds, have a flushed face or AIDS. Remember large doses may cause vomiting.

Comfrey: *Symphytum officindale*

Uses: Wounds, insect bites, burns, poison ivy, inflammation, bruised and damaged joints and muscles

Comfrey's nickname is knitbone. The allantoin in Comfrey actually causes cells to proliferate, making comfrey the most recommended herbal remedy for skin disorders and healing wounds. The root has a higher content of allantoin than the leaves. The leaves are more astringent and has more anti-inflammatory properties. Comfrey is rich in calcium, potassium, phosphorus, and vitamins A and C.[3]

Because of Comfrey's high mucilage content, the highest of any herb, it is good where moistening and lubrications is needed.

Before Plaster of Paris, cloths were dipped in a tea of Comfrey root, wrapped around the injured limb and left to harden as a cast.

At one time Comfrey was one of the most recommended herbs for internal use. It was recommended for ulcers, bronchial irritation, pneumonia, and inflammations of the stomach. It was eaten as a potherb and is one of the few vegetarian sources of B12.

Comfrey is no longer recommended internally because of possible liver damage and cancer. It is still considered safe for external application.

Even though you cannot take tinctures and teas of Comfrey internally they are valuable as a soak or compress for injuries and skin irritations when an oil would not be appropriate.

There are 2 cases of liver damage by individuals taking excessive amounts of Comfrey over a long length of time.

---

[3] Growing and Using the Healing Herbs, page 118

Some herbalists still recommend Comfrey as long as it is not taken internally for over 3 months.

Test animals were fed large doses of Comfrey for 2 years before liver cancer developed.

Cancer authority Bruce Ames, PH.D chairman of the biochemistry department at the University of California at Berkeley compared the cancer risk of one cup of Comfrey tea to the same as one peanut butter sandwich, 1/3 the risk of eating one raw mushroom, ½ half the risk of one diet soda containing saccharin, 1/100 the risk of a standard glass of beer or wine.[4]

Leaves can be harvested all year round but are best right before they bloom. The roots are to be harvested in the fall or early spring.

Although herb books may say that you can grow Comfrey in full sun that does not mean Texas. It will do better in partial shade in an area you can keep well watered. Comfrey likes rich moist soil.

Propagate Comfrey by planting 2" pieces of the root upright in a pot with the tip showing at the top. It usually takes 3-4 weeks for the root to leaf out.

See Chapter for Comfrey oil, lotions, lip balms and salves beginning page 79

Comfrey does not have antiseptic properties so should not be used before cleaning the wound. Do not apply to major wounds before they are healed on the inside. Comfrey can cause the skin to heal over leaving infection inside the wound.

---

[4] 100 Healing Herbs

Echinacea: Purpurea, E. Angustifolia, E. Pallida *The Purple Coneflower*

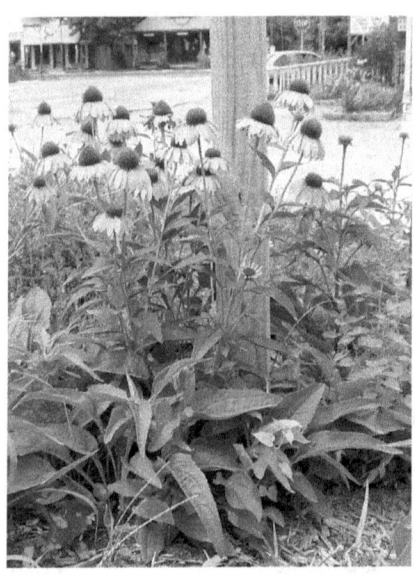

If you are allergic to ragweed or other plants in the Asteraceae (daisy) family avoid Echinacea.

Echinacea is one of the most studied herbs in herbal medicine. Native to North America was widely used by the American Indians. The Omaha-Ponca Indians chewed the roots of the Echinacea for tooth pain. The juice from the roots was used to treat burns and wounds. The Cheyenne brewed a tea from the roots and leaves to soothe sore throats, gums and sores of the mouth. The roots of Echinacea was used to treat snakebites.

Today it is recommended as an immune system builder. Studies show that it increases the antibody response, elevating interferon levels for fighting viruses, and stimulates the white blood cells to work harder against infections.[5] Research shows that taking Echinacea on a daily basis does not prevent the cold or flu.

Echinacea is recommended to shorten the duration of colds and flu, and to treat wounds.

---

[5] National Geographic's Guide to Medicinal Herbs

Elderberry: *Sambucus canadenis or s. nigra*

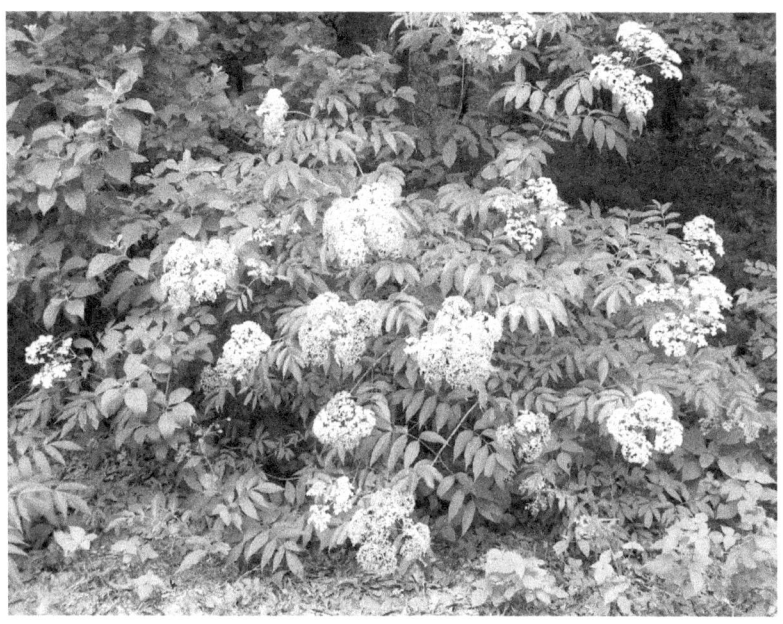

Elderberry is a common bush growing wild all over East Texas and other southern states. You will usually find it growing in the ditches or other wet areas. It is an old folk remedy at least 2500 years old. It is being imported from Israel, of all places, and sold in the health food stores under the name Sambucol. Dried Elderberries are coming from Croatia.

This centuries old folk remedy for colds and flu has been verified with research by Dr. Madeline Mumcuoglu. The flowers and berries contain 2 chemicals that prevent the flu virus from invading throat cells and replicating themselves in the body.

The flu virus has tiny spikes that pierce the cells in your body. Elderberries have a protein that coats the spikes, preventing the spikes from piercing the cell membranes. The flu virus spikes also have an enzyme that breaks down the cell walls. The Elderberry neutralizes this enzyme. Elderberries enhance the immune system and is good for other respiratory infections.

In 1992 a flu outbreak occurred in southern Israel. Half the residents were given an elderberry formula of 4 tablespoon a day. The other half, were given Tylenol and other cold formulas. 90 percent of the Elderberry group felt better in 3 days while the other group felt better in 6 days. A few years ago, at the first sign of the flu (sore throat, fever and hurting to the bone), I took Elderberry syrup, no aspirins, Echinacea and went to bed. I was well the next day. I didn't feel great, but I didn't have the flu.

People make the mistake of taking aspirins at the first sign of fever. **Wrong,** !!!. At the first sign of a virus the body heats up to kill the virus. When you take aspirin to bring down your fever, you are fighting against your body's defense system trying to heal itself. Don't take aspirin unless you fever is over 102°f degrees, or unless instructed to do so by your physician. These instructions apply to adults only and not to children or the elderly.

Elderberry leaves can be used for bruises, sprains, wounds and tumors. To make an Elderberry ointment, bruise three parts fresh elder leaves with 6 parts oil and cook on low heat until the leaves are crisp. Add beeswax. Older herbals will use Vaseline. Strain and store in a cool, dark place. The leaves and stems are poisonous taken internally.

The Elderflowers or berries can be used for upper respiratory tract inflammations and rheumatism.

The flowers are prepared as a tea. Pour a cup of boiling water over 2 teaspoons of dried or fresh elder flowers. Steep for 10 minutes. This should be drunk hot 3 times a day. It would combine well with peppermint.

Start looking for the elderberries in your area. During the month of June you can see the tiny white flowers that make up a big white umbrella shaped flower the size of a saucer. These flowers will turn into BB size berries.

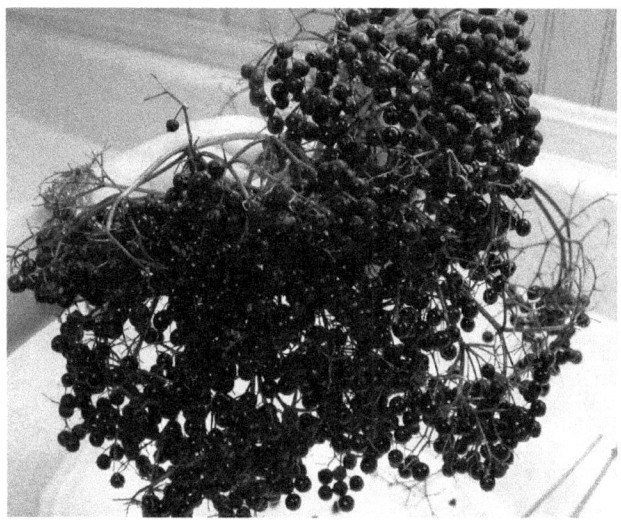

The berries are ready to harvest when they turn black in August or September, depending on the weather.

Elderberries are available dried.

Recipes for Elderberry Syrup on page 36

Frankincense and Myrrh: Boswellia carteri and Commiphora myrrha

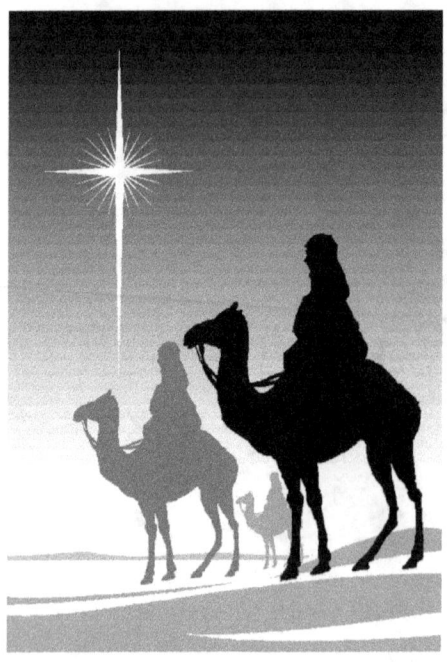

> *Frankincense and Myrrh-gifts to the baby Jesus- were being used thousands of years before the birth of Christ in Egypt for anointing and healing the sick.*

Matthew 2: 11- KJV: And when they were come into the house, they saw the young child with Mary his mother and fell down and worshipped him: and when they had opened their treasures, they presented unto him gifts, gold, Frankincense and Myrrh.

We all know what gold is. What about Frankincense and Myrrh? What we know is much like the children in the Christmas play. The 3 wise men each had one word to say. The first child said "gold". The second child said "Myrrh". The third child proudly pronounced "Frank sent this".

Frankincense and Myrrh-gifts to the baby Jesus- were being used thousands of years before the birth of Christ in Egypt for anointing and healing the sick. It was also used religiously in the Egyptian,

Greek and Roman temples.

Medical scrolls indicate the Egyptians had a high success rate treating 81 different diseases using essential oils such as Myrrh.

Frankincense and Myrrh are used in cosmetics for aging skin.

Myrrh was used in embalming the dead and Frankincense is used in the production of incense.

Frankincense and Myrrh are resins from small trees. Frankincense is grown in Arabia, Africa, and China. Myrrh is native to Arabia, Somalia, Ethiopia, and other North African countries.

Frankincense and Myrrh is harvest much like the syrup of maple trees. A small slit is cut in the bark and the sap is collected.

Frankincense sap or resin is called tears.

The resin from Myrrh is called pearls.

Frankincense and Myrrh are first mentioned in the Bible when the tabernacle is being built in Exodus 30: 22-38.

"Then the Lord said to Moses, take the following fine spices: 500 shekels of liquid Myrrh, half as much of fragrant Cinnamon, 250 shekels of fragrant Cane, 500 shekels of Cassia-all according to the sanctuary shekel- and a hin of olive oil. Make these into a sacred anointing oil, a fragrant blend, the work of a perfumer. It will be the sacred anointing oil." Exodus 30: 22-25. If you read the whole passage this blend was **only for the temple and priest and strictly forbidden to be used by any one else.**

What you smell while you sleep can influence how you dream.

Essential oils of all kinds are now being rediscovered by today's scientist and doctors. Frankincense is being researched and used therapeutically in European hospitals. Frankincense is being studied as an immune stimulator, its ability to increase oxygen around the pineal gland and pituitary gland and help alleviate manic depressive symptoms.

Frankincense was burned as incense in temples of many religions. Frankincense causes a person to breathe deeper and slower which is good for meditation and prayer. Frankincense was burned in public gatherings and in homes to purify the air. Many essential oils kill airborne diseases such as Staphylococcus aureus and Streptococcus pyogenes within hours. More essential oils which were proven in a clinical study are Clove, Lavender, Lemon, Marjoram, Peppermint, Niaouli, Pine, Rosemary, and Thyme. Frankincense effects the respiratory system, being effective for ailments such as asthma and bronchitis. It is a balsamic agent (soothing) for colds, chills, congestion, etc.

Frankincense may also be used as a compress for inflammations. The essential oil can be sprinkled on gauze, flannel, etc. and laid on top of the inflamed site. The most effective way to use essential oils are to use steam inhalation. This may be accomplished by sprinkling essential oils into hot water and inhaling the steam, or using an inexpensive humidifier. I run a cool water humidifier in my home and sprinkle essential oils on a tissue and lay across the opening to purify and to scent the air. Or you can simmer water on the stovetop with essential oils. Try a diffuser. I would encourage people that are using candles to scent the air to try one of these methods.

So many people worry about smoke from cigarette smokers and don't even think about the candles. Besides the wax being released into the air, most candles are scented with synthetic scents which are petroleum based.

Steam inhalation is most effective for breaking up congestion and coughs.

Myrrh is recognized for its ability to help with infections of the skin and throat, regenerate skin tissue and its effectiveness in preventing bacterial growth. It is being used for asthma, bronchitis, decongestions of the prostrate glands and normalizing hyperthyroid problems. Myrrh tincture has been shown to be effective as a mouthwash for sore teeth and gums and taken internally for spongy gums and loose teeth. Myrrh increases circulation and increases activity of the white blood cells to fight infection.

Myrrh can be used in steam inhalation therapy and as compresses as described for Frankincense. Myrrh is used in steam inhalation as a cough expectorant.

Myrrh is especially effective for mouth sores and canker sores. A dropper full of tincture of myrrh (tinctures are different than a bottle of essential oil) can be place on a sterile piece of gauze on placed on the canker sore 10-15 minutes 4 times a day. Or a less effective method would be to add a dropper full of tincture of Myrrh in 4 oz. of water and swish in the mouth 4 times a day.

Mild Hypothyroidism can be treated with 1/8-1/4 teaspoons of tincture of myrrh 3 times a day. I emphasize mild, because hypothyroidism can be a serious condition and if you are under a doctor's care don't stop your treatments. Definitely do not use on a child unless you have a qualified person to help you.

Essential oils are effective being inhaled or massaged into the skin. They do not need to be ingested. Essential oils applied to the feet will be throughout the body including the hair in 20 minutes.

Bible students have seen in the gifts symbols of Christ's identity and what he would accomplish. Gold was a gift for a king, Frankincense, a gift for deity, Myrrh, a spice for a person who was going to die. I believe Our God provides us with real gifts and not just symbols. Maybe these gifts were God's provisions to protect the frail human body of baby Jesus.

Ginger: Zinger official

Ginger is a stimulating herb and often used in herbal preparations as a carrier helping to move the other herbs through the body.

Ginger can be compared to Dramamine in its effectiveness for motion sickness and morning sickness and will not make you sleepy. I use it when sinus drainage makes me nauseous.

For motion sickness, 1500 milligrams is recommended 30 minutes before travel. Ginger capsules can be used, or a 12 oz glass of real Ginger Ale or Ginger tea. I prefer the ginger candy. I can keep it in my purse ready when I need it.

A hot foot bath of Ginger tea, may stop the onset of a cold, warm up cold feet and stop body pains. A cup of hot ginger tea will increase circulation warming up toes, feet and hands and has virus killing compounds that will help ward of the cold or flu. A gargle of Ginger tea or Ginger tincture, will help a sore throat. A compress of Ginger tea placed over the throat can stop sore throat pain.

A Ginger compress can ease the pain of arthritis and sore joints. Rub Ginger juice on the skin, or dilute the essential oil of Ginger.

A Ginger compress over the lungs can help break up congestion. Ginger tea is my favorite for clearing up mucus.

The New England Journal of Medicine reports that Ginger reduces cholesterol, helps lower blood pressure and prevents internal blood clots.

The root of Ginger is not boiled when making a tea, except when making Ginger Ale. See recipes pages 30-31

Precautions: May cause heartburn, pregnant women should not take more than 1 gram of powdered Ginger a day, do not take large amounts of Ginger if you are taking blood thinners.

Growing Ginger:
Take a piece or fresh root that has at least 2 eyes. Plant in loose, rich soil with good drainage, 3 inches deep and 12 inches apart. The temperature must be kept a minimum of 70°F constantly. The shoots should pop up in about 2 weeks. The roots or rhizomes should be ready to harvest in 9 months.

Hops: Humulus lupulus

Hops, widely known as an ingredient in beer, is also one of the most used herbs for insomnia and now used for pain and inflammation. It can be drank as a tea but it is very bitter. It is mostly taken in capsules or tinctures.

Hops has a relaxing effect on the central nervous system. It eases tension and anxiety, and is useful for treating restlessness, and headache caused by tension. Caution, if beer gives you a headache, hops may also.
A hops sleeping pillow is an old folk remedy used by King George III, Abraham Lincoln, and the Prince of Wales.

Dolls stuffed with Hops and Lavender and even Dill Seed were used to help children sleep.

Native Americans drank hops tea as a sedative. They heated the strobiles in a bag and applied to the face for tooth aches.

Caution: Do not use with marked depression. Do not use internally if pregnant, nursing or have breast cancer. Hops may contain chemicals similar to estrogen.

Special extracts of hops are standardized for pain relief and as an anti-inflammatory without the dangerous side effects of NSAIDS.

The standardized extract have removed the sleep inducing properties and the estrogen like properties making it safe for most people.

The 2 brands I know of are Purluxen and Vinoprin.

Hops prefer deep damp soil. It can take full sun if plenty of water is provided. The roots are hardy to -35 degrees and prefer soil with a PH of 6.0-7.0. They will die back in the winter and come back the next spring. Mulch the plants heavily before winter. Choose 3-4 vines and train around a trellis or a fence. Cut the remaining vines to the ground. After the first year hop vines can grow over 6 inches a day. Mid to late summer, green blossoms will appear. They will look like little miniature pinecones. They are ready to harvest in late summer or early fall. The hop fruit is called strobiles. They are ready to harvest when they are dry and turning yellow.

Strobiles are dried in the shade and should be stored away from heat and sunlight.

The aroma of hops will become concentrated with age.

The vines can be braided into wreaths or baskets.

Mexican Marigold Mint: Tagetes lucida

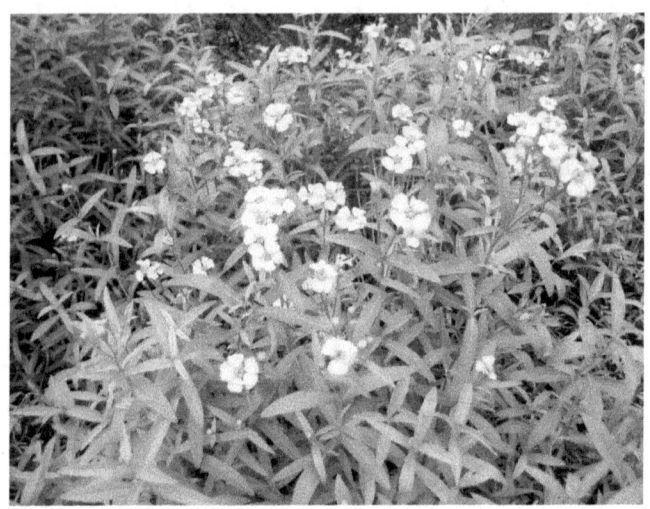

I don't know why I fell in love with this particular licorice scented herb. I was never particularly overly fond of the scent of licorice. There were certainly many licorice scented herbs to choose from, Licorice, Anise, Tarragon, Fennel, Chervil, Anise Hyssop also called Licorice mint, and Hoja Santa. I just couldn't breathe in that delicious aroma deep enough. The scent was intoxicating and addicting. I needed to inhale it and taste it. I chewed the leaves hoping to capture the aroma and satisfy my sudden addiction to that scent. That however, does not work. The only way to capture and enjoy this licorice aroma would be in the kitchen.

The first obvious choice would be an herbal tea. I am from Texas. In Texas, tea means iced tea, not hot tea. Since I first discovered and fell in love with herbs, I have tried unsuccessfully to develop a taste for hot tea.

Most of the herb books, tea is always hot tea. Steep a pot of hot tea, invite friends over for a cup of hot tea. I have spent years trying different combinations of herbs to find a hot tea that I like. Then it dawned on me. I don't have to drink hot herbal tea, just make herbal tea like I normally make iced tea. Then a whole new world of herbal teas opened up to me when I started making iced, herbal tea. I simply add a bunch of MMM leaves to my black tea and steep together.

I learned Mexican Marigold Mint is also called Texas Tarragon, and was used as a substitute for French Tarragon. French Tarragon cannot withstand the heat and humidity of Texas. Mexican Marigold Mint loves the heat and grows just great in Texas. This little East Texas girl had no idea what Tarragon was or how it was used in the kitchen. I don't think I knew anyone in my circle of friends who had ever heard or used French Tarragon. The word "French" was a dead give a-way right there. That sounded just a little too fancy for me. Our idea of foreign food is Tex-Mex. So I gave up the culinary aspects of this herb for the time being.

There was not much information about Mexican Marigold Mint in the many herb books that I own. It seems as most of the herb books are about herbs from the Old World, Europe. Most of the herb books are written by authors from Europe or authors gathering their information from those books that are written by authors from Europe.

Mexican Marigold Mint is a New World herb, native to Mexico and Guatemala. So I set out find out as much as I could about this little Mexican herb.

Its' foliage is used in teas, seasonings and medical purposes such as calming stomachs and nerves, colds and colic. It has a reputation for curing a hangover. There was also reference for it being used for malaria and crushing the leaves as a poultice for snake bites.

Mexican Marigold Mint has quite a reputation in Mexico. It goes by cloud plant, sweet mace, winter or Mexican tarragon, mint scented marigold, root beer plant, and yerba anis.

The Tarahumara Indians of Chihuahua and the Huichol Indians of Jalisco and Nayarit use it in their religious rituals.

It's reputation goes all the way back to the 16th century recorded by the Spanish explorers. It was supposedly one of the herbs powdered and blew into the faces of the sacrificial victims of the Aztecs right before their hearts were ripped out of their chests.

Don't confuse Mexican Marigold Mint with Calendula Marigold, (Calendula officinalis L.). Even though the European herbalists called Calendula, Marigold or Pot Marigold, it is not kin to Mexican Marigold Mint.

Mexican Marigold Mint is however kin to the French Marigold.

Mexican Marigold Mint blooms in the fall. Like most herbs, it requires well drained soil and little fertilizer. It will take full sun but will tolerate partial shade. Once established it is drought tolerant. It is considered a perennial as long as it doesn't go below 20 degrees f. in your area. It will re-seed itself. It can be propagated by dividing a clump in the spring, or rooting the cuttings. It will get 2-3 feet tall and expand about 2 feet. The herb books will tell you that 2 plants are plenty. Those authors are obviously not addicted to Mexican Marigold Mint.

It holds up well as a cut flower and is used in dried flower arrangements and dried as an addition to potpourri.

Back to the kitchen. See pages starting at 29 for recipes

17 Measurements and Ratios

These are approximate, some essential oils are thicker than others, and droppers are larger or smaller.

½ ml = 8 drops = 1/8 dram
5/8 ml = 10 drops = 1/8 teaspoon = 1/6 dram
1 ml = 30 drops
1 ¼ ml = 20 drops = ¼ teaspoon = 1/3 dram
2 ½ ml = 40 drops = ½ teaspoon =2/3 dram
 5 ml = 150 drops = 1 teaspoon = 1/3 tablespoon = 1 1/3 dram
10 ml = 300 drops = 2 teaspoons =
15 ml = 1 tablespoon = 3 teaspoons = 4 drams
30 ml = 1 fluid ounce
500 ml = 500 grams = ½ kilo= 16 fluid ounces = 1 pint
1000 ml = 1 litre

1 tablespoon = 3 teaspoons
4 tablespoons = ¼ cup= 2 fluid ounces
5 1/3 tablespoons = 1/3 cup
8 tablespoons = ½ cup = 4 fluid ounces
12 tablespoons = ¾ cup = 6 fluid ounces
16 tablespoons = 1 cup = 8 fluid ounces
1 fluid ounce = 2 tablespoons
1 cup = ½ pint = 8 fluid ounces
2 cups = 1 pint = 16 fluid ounces
4 cups = 2 pints = 1 quart =32 fluid ounces
4 quarts = 1 gallon = 128 fluid ounces

¼ teaspoon = 1.25 ml
½ teaspoon = 2.5 ml
1 teaspoon = 5 ml
1 tablespoon = 15 ml
¼ cup = 60 ml
1/3 cup = 80 ml
½ cup= 120 ml
1 cup = 235 ml

Ratios of Carrier Oils to Essential Oils:

There are different opinions and some oils are more aggressive than others. These are ratios are for using therapeutic grade essential oils. Some people are more sensitive than others and you need to reduce by ½ for children, the elderly and pregnant women.

Herbs for Health and Healing
1 drop as a perfume
1 drop to scent a handkerchief or stationary
2 drops to fabric to scent a drawer
2 drops on 1 tablespoon of salt as a smelling salt
2 drops for ½ cup of water to use as a compress
6 drops in 1 oz of herbal skin cream or aloe vera gel or juice
12 drops in 1 ounce of massage oil
12 drops in 1 ounce of salve
24 drops in ¼ cup of salt per bath or 1 ounce of bath oil

Flower Road Natural Therapies
Physical effect: 30 ml or 1 ounce of carrier oil plus 1 ml or 30 drops of essential oil
Scent only: 30 ml or 1 ounce of carrier oil plus 10 drops of essential oil

Young Living Essential Oils
15-30 drops per carrier oil as a general rule
Equal parts of carrier oil to essential oil for some essential oils
1 part essential oil to 4 parts essential oil for more aggressive essential oils

Ratios for Teas, Tinctures, Oils

Teas:

Hot Infusion: leaves, flowers and green stems
1 teaspoon of dried herb or 3 teaspoons of fresh per 1 cup of boiling water, steep for 10-15 minutes

Decoctions: hard and woody ,roots, hard seeds, barks, nuts, rhizomes
1 teaspoon of dried herb or 3 teaspoons of fresh herbs brought to a boil and simmered 10-15 minutes.

Tinctures:
4 oz. of dried herb or 8 oz. of fresh herb to 1 pint of 60-80 proof Vodka or other alcohol.
Shake 2 x a day for 6 weeks, strain and bottle

Herbal Oils:
4 tablespoons (2 oz.) of dried herb or ½ cup of fresh herb to 2 cups of vegetable oil. Let set in dark, place for 3 days, strain and bottle adding ½ teaspoon of Vitamin E and essential oil of choice.
Optional: Simmer over low heat (160°F) for 1 hour.

Salves and Ointments:
Add 1 oz. of beeswax per 1 cup of herbal oil.

Bath Tea:
1 quart of boiling water to ½ cup of dried herb or 1 cup of fresh herb

Carolyn Gibson

THE AUTHOR

Carolyn Gibson LMT, MI and CE Provider has been a registered massage therapist since 1996. She fell in love with herbs in the early 70's and has been studying them since that time.

Her and her husband Gerald Gibson are owners of Dogwood Gardens Organic Farm, certified organic since 1991.

They started out growing medical herbs and now grow Wheatgrass only.

Other Books by Carolyn Gibson
On Amazon

How to be a Good Wife
Trigger Point Made Easy

Books on Kindle
All About Wheatgrass
Unique DIY Centerpieces

Carolyn Gibson

www.ingramcontent.com/pod-product-compliance
Lightning Source LLC
Chambersburg PA
CBHW070427290526
45791CB00005B/1873